IMMUNE BOOSTERS

THE SCIENCE ON SUPPLEMENTS AND IMMUNITY

DOMINICK BOSCO

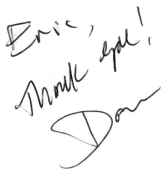

Eric,
Thank you!
Dom

ALSO BY DOMINICK BOSCO

Bedlam: A Year In The Life Of A Mental Hospital

What People Who Take Vitamin C Know That You Don't

Alone With The Devil (with Ronald Markman, MD)

Confessions Of A Medical Heretic (for Robert S. Mendelsohn, MD)

The People's Guide To Vitamins And Minerals

Wild Pizza

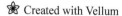 Created with Vellum

For my family

CONTENTS

SUPPLEMENTS MIGHT HELP— EMPHASIS ON "MIGHT"

The purpose of this book is to share information about the scientific research on supplements—vitamins, herbs, and other nutrients—and how they *might possibly* help strengthen the body's defenses against infection and inflammation.

I hasten to emphasize the words *might possibly.*

At times like this, with a deadly virus in the air, it's natural to interpret "might possibly" as "will definitely." Don't do it. That is not the intent of this book. The intent is to report what I found when I delved into the scientific research on how nutritional and herbal supplements affect the immune system.

Because I am not qualified to prescribe or make therapeutic recommendations, I have made no recommendations for which supplements to take or not take. Nothing in this book should be interpreted as a prescription for what will work for you or me or anyone else.

Nutritional and herbal supplements might help fortify our defenses, but they are not the solution to the coronavirus or COVID-19. At some point—we pray soon—medical research will develop successful treatments and an effective vaccine. Until then, avoiding contact with the virus is our best bet. That's not a disclaimer, that's a fact.

The book began with communication between my family and me regarding supplements that might possibly:

1.) Help strengthen our immune defenses against viral infections, and

2.) Reduce inflammation in hopes of lowering the likelihood of runaway inflammation in the event of an infection.

We began exchanging links to articles and scientific papers and, before long, I found myself immersed in online research.

I approached the scientific literature with a specific purpose: to find research on how vitamins, minerals, herbs, and other supplements affect the immune system. But there's a lot of research out there and reporting all of it, or even most of it, would require a book many times this size.

So I tried to achieve the same balance as the research itself. I didn't report every positive or every negative finding. But if the preponderance of the research I saw seemed to find a positive effect, that is reflected in the chapter.

For most of the supplements there was at least one review paper that described results of prior research. So it was possible to get an idea of the prevailing scientific opinion on whether the supplement was a net plus, minus, or neutral when it came to supporting the immune system.

There is very little supplement research that directly addresses the new coronavirus and COVID-19.

But there is a lot of research that scientifically addresses the question of whether certain supplements and herbs can support the healthy function of the immune system to fight off an infection or come through it faster, with reduced symptoms.

Supplements are not cures. They're not a sure thing. They don't provide invulnerability against infection. They are never a substitute for qualified medical care. The best they can do is strengthen the body's natural defenses. They can't promise more against a virus than *maybe* ever-so-slightly nudging the odds towards our favor. Sometimes, as it is with other things in life, that can be enough.

VITAMINS & MINERALS

1

VITAMIN A

In 1928 two of the medical doctors studying vitamin A called it "the anti-inflammation vitamin."[1] We know even more than they did almost 100 years ago, and the name still applies.

In fact, we might add to the name and also refer to vitamin A as "the immunity vitamin." In addition to its role maintaining vision and growth, vitamin A is vital to what scientists now refer to as the "front lines of defense against pathogen invasion," the mucous and epithelial tissues. These tissues require vitamin A to grow, mature, function, and survive.

Vitamin A is essential to the layer of mucus covering the mucous membranes. Without enough vitamin A, these critical immune tissues in the skin, digestive tract, respiratory tract, genitourinary system, eyes, and soft tissues for all practical purposes shrink and die and leave our defenses dramatically weakened. [2]

. . .

Crucial To Protection From Respiratory Disease

Studies of tuberculosis demonstrate that the disease proliferates where dietary vitamin A is lower. Vitamin A has shown promise treating diseases that infect the body through the respiratory system, such as measles and pneumonia, and also in infectious digestive diseases. The World Health Organization has recommended children in developing countries receive high doses of vitamin A to reduce the incidence and mortality of these diseases. [3]

But there is evidence that vitamin A deficiency also exists in developed countries. A study of American infants discovered deficiencies in two-thirds of infants under 3 months old and in one-quarter of 4-6-month old infants. [4]

There's more. We say an army marches on its stomach, but our immune system army that defends us against everything from the common cold to COVID-19 marches on vitamin A. All crucial immune organs require constant dietary intake of vitamin A—and not just as a foot soldier, but as a general, regulating and directing vital immune functions such as macrophages, neutrophils, and killer T cells. Yes, and cytokines, too. Vitamin A is critical to the cells that regulate inflammation. [5]

Vitamin A Supplements Against Inflammation

Vitamin A deficiency induces inflammation and makes existing inflammatory states worse. Supplementation helps. This has been demonstrated in animal and human studies.[6]

In human studies, high dietary levels of vitamin A reduce highly inflammatory cytokines. In one such study 28 overweight young women were given 25,000 IU of vitamin A per day for 4 months. A similar group was given placebo and a third group of non-obese women also received vitamin A. Inflammatory cytokines were measured in all women at the outset and then again at the end of the study. The obese women, as expected, had initially higher levels of inflammatory cytokines. In both the obese and non-obese women, vitamin A supplements significantly reduced inflammatory cytokines. [7]

It's also been shown in a study with children infected with respiratory syncytial virus that children with low levels of vitamin A had more severe illness. [8]

Scientists believe that lower levels of vitamin A found during infectious diseases create a vicious cycle. The infection and inflammation cause more vitamin A to be used up in tissue defense and repair, causing an even worse deficiency—and making the infection and the tissue-destructive inflammation still worse! [9]

A study of people with COPD (chronic obstructive pulmonary disease) found that there was a direct relationship between vitamin A levels and the extent of airway obstruction. COPD patients with higher intake of vitamin A experienced less difficulty breathing. [10]

Prevailing Scientific Opinion: Deficiency weakens the immune system. Adequate intake supports immunity.

2

B VITAMINS

I DIDN'T USUALLY THINK OF THE B VITAMINS AS BEING involved in immunity and inflammation. But in the interest of thoroughness, I did what I expected to be a cursory search for scientific evidence that B vitamins could somehow help.

Wow, was I surprised.

The doorway to understanding the importance of B vitamins to the immune system is through their established effects on the nervous system. Scientists looking into how B vitamins affect mood and other psychological states have taken the position that the B vitamins exert their affect by modulating inflammation. [1]

That was news to me. It's not the purpose of this book to make or break the case that inflammation causes depression, anxiety, or other mental problems. But just the fact that scientists view B vitamins as crucial to the immune system and reducing inflammation—well, after seeing that, I knew this chapter had to explore what role each of the B vitamins actually might play in helping our immune system fight off viruses and suppress inflammation. With that in mind:

B1, Thiamin, works as an antioxidant and modulates the immune system's cytokine response. A deficiency triggers cytokine release and leads to neuro-inflammation and neuron cell death. [2]

B2, Riboflavin, activates a major part of the immune system's defenses against infection. A deficiency weakens the immune system and promotes inflammation. [3]

An animal study found that riboflavin headed off cytokines by inhibiting the release of a signaling protein that stimulates inflammation. I found this study interesting because the doctors were *specifically* investigating riboflavin as a potential therapy for septic shock, or cytokine storm. In their paper they referred to several other animal studies showing riboflavin ability to inhibit inflammation and prevent animals' death from septic shock.[4]

B3, Niacin, dampens inflammation by down-regulating cytokines and preventing oxidative damage. Nicotinamide, another form of the vitamin, counteracted the inflammatory effects of a special diet in animals. [5] A study of airline pilots found that diets high in niacin, whole grains, and low in red meat had a protective effect against DNA damage from exposure to ionizing radiation. [6]

. . .

Pantothenic Acid intake was found to affect low-grade chronic inflammation in men and women aged 40 or older. Increased inflammation seemed to accompany low dietary levels. [7]

B6, Pyridoxal-5-phosphate, suppresses oxidative damage and cytokine stimulation. A deficiency weakens the immune system's ability to fight off infections and control inflammation. Many diseases resulting from B6 deficiency are associated with chronic inflammation. A study of over 2000 adults found that low levels of B6 were associated with higher levels of inflammation. [8] [9]

B6 supplements (100 mg/day) for 12 weeks significantly reduced inflammatory cytokines in people with rheumatoid arthritis. [10]

Folic Acid inhibits cytokine activation and regulates the immune response. A deficiency weakens the immune system and disrupts regulation of cytokines. [11] Folic acid supplements (400 mcg/day) for 12 months reduced inflammatory cytokine levels and significantly improved cognitive performance in 77 elderly people with mild impairment. [12]

B12, cobalamin, regulates the immune system. A deficiency weakens the immune system and increases cytokines. [13] In a study of 364 adults and children, low levels of B12 were linked to higher levels of inflammatory cytokines. [14]

. . .

Choline also plays a role in regulating cytokines. Several animal studies have demonstrated that a choline-rich diet and/or choline treatment has a protective effect in sepsis. In humans, increased choline decreases levels of homocysteine, a significant marker for inflammation. [15]

Inositol appears to regulate one of the primary inflammatory cytokines and has already been tested as a treatment for respiratory distress syndrome in newborns—which resembles cytokine storm— and found effective in reducing inflammation and increasing survival. [16] Several studies in animals have demonstrated that inositol deficiency predisposes to cytokine storm. And inositol has recently been proposed as a possible treatment for cytokine storm caused by COVID-19. [17]

Biotin deficiency increases inflammatory cytokines and weakens the immune system. [18] [19]

You could write an entire book on each of the B vitamins, so getting even a flavor of all the research out there in this limited space would be impossible. Based on the research cited here, the B vitamins are critical to the healthy function of the immune system.

Prevailing Scientific Opinion: Deficiency weakens the

immune system and promotes inflammation. Adequate intake helps control inflammation.

VITAMIN C

THERE'S A REASON VITAMIN C IS THE MOST POPULAR vitamin supplement on earth: there's a LOT of research on it, the vast majority of it positive. This is not the place to go into all the proven benefits of vitamin C. We're going to limit this to two questions:

1.) Is there scientific evidence that vitamin C can help strengthen natural defenses to viral infections?

2.) Is there evidence that vitamin C can reduce inflammation or improve related processes or biomarkers?

The answer to both questions is yes.

The Wuhan Study Of Fatal Cases

On April 3, 2020, the American Thoracic Society reported a new study attempting to identify the biomarkers of COVID-19 patients most likely to perish from the infection. [1] The Chinese and American doctors looked at the medical records of 85 patients who died from the infection. In addition to the usual characteristics reported all over the news—mostly males over 50 with chronic diseases such as diabetes, heart disease and high blood pressure—they also found 81% of the patients had low levels of eosinophils when admitted to the hospital. [2]

Eosinophils are white blood cells. They're supposed to go up during an infection, not down. They're critical to effective immunity.

What does this have to do with vitamin C?

Vitamin C helps regulate eosinophils. It elevates them when they're low and lowers them when they're too high, as they can be in asthma. In animal studies, vitamin C prevented the dramatic depletion of eosinophils by alcohol, [3] and heat. [4]

Would vitamin C have helped the people in the Wuhan study? Judging from their pre-existing chronic diseases, their nutritional status was probably not so great. So adding some vitamin C to their diets *before they got sick* might have helped, but whether it would have made the difference, no one can say.

Vitamin C and Flu

We already know that vitamin C can help prevent, shorten the duration, and reduce the severity of the common cold.[5] But what about flu?

There have been studies where people with flu infections were given vitamin C. In one such study 252 students ages 18 to 30 were given 1 gram of vitamin C three times a day. If they reported symptoms of respiratory infections, the dose was increased to 1 gram per hour for six hours, then back to 1 gram three times a day. The people who received vitamin C had 85 percent fewer cold and flu symptoms than those who were given standard over-the-counter remedies instead of vitamin C.[6]

An animal study found that vitamin C stimulates antiviral immune responses when given early on in an influenza infection through increased production of antiviral interferon α and β. Whereas all of the animals who were initially deficient in vitamin C succumbed to the infection—even though they were given more vitamin C on the second day of the infection— all of the animals who had adequate levels of vitamin C *from the beginning* survived. The lungs of the animals who died had 10-15 times more virus and more damage from out-of-control immune response. In other words, cytokine storm. The study's conclusion: damage through the growth of influenza viruses can be prevented when vitamin C concentration is high enough at the initial stage of viral infection. If it is not sufficient, however, the progress of the influenza infection cannot be prevented.[7]

Intravenous Vitamin C and Sepsis (Cytokine Storm)

In animal studies, vitamin C reduces pro-inflammatory cytokines and boosts anti-inflammatory cytokines.[8] [9] There are also studies where vitamin C was given intravenously to people with sepsis. It's not really within the scope of this book to cover such extraordinary treatments. The chances you or your family could talk the attending physicians at the hospital to give you intravenous vitamin C are probably small, unless the physician was remarkably up-to-date on the research.

In one study, 47 severely ill ICU sepsis patients were treated with intravenous vitamin C, thiamine, and hydrocortisone and compared to 47 patients who did not receive the treatment. Mortality was 8.5% in the treatment group and 40.4% in the untreated group. The Sepsis-Related Organ Failure Assessment (SOFA) score decreased in all the treated patients. Not a single person in the treated group suffered increasing organ failure. [10]

In another study, ICU sepsis patients who received intravenous vitamin C immediately saw their SOFA scores and their biochemical markers of inflammation drop. Their conclusion was that the treatment was safe, could reduce inflammation, and help prevent organ failure and tissue damage.[11]

Vitamin C Supplements and Ultramarathoners

Probably the best indication we have that supplementing with vitamin C *before* an event that stimulates the production of cytokines is the experiment done with runners training for a 90 km ultramarathon. One group of runners were supplemented with 500 mg of vitamin C per day for a week before the race, one group received 1500 mg per day for a week before the race, and one group received no vitamin C at all. Cytokines and cortisol were dramatically and significantly lower in the 1500 mg/day runners compared to the 500 mg/day and zero mg/day runners. [12]

Vitamin C and Pneumonia

Vitamin C can also help prevent and successfully treat pneumonia. A review of previous research found that there was an 80% or greater reduction in cases of pneumonia in people supplemented with vitamin C. This same review reported lower mortality and reduced symptoms in the most severely ill elderly patients supplemented with vitamin C. A study of adults in the former Soviet Union found that higher doses of vitamin C resulted in a faster recovery. [13]

A study in China found that vitamin C inhibited pro-inflammatory cytokines and oxidative damage to lung tissue in people with severe community-acquired pneumonia. [14]

How Much Vitamin C?

Linus Pauling, the only person to ever win two unshared Nobel Prizes, each in a different category, recommended taking at least 2 grams a day. Dr. Albert Szent-Gyorgi, 1937 Nobel laureate in medicine, who won for his work on vitamin C, confided to Pauling that he took 1000 mg per day.

Straight up or extended release?

Does it make a difference? One study found that extended release dosing smoothed out fluctuations in blood concentrations but the end effect of the differences would probably not be significant. [15]

Prevailing Scientific Opinion: Deficiency seriously weakens the immune system. Research on supplementing above RDA suggests some benefit.

VITAMIN D

VITAMIN D IS A MAJOR PLAYER IN THE IMMUNE WARS: IT'S one of the natural substances that not only has anti-inflammatory powers, but it can also help fight off viruses, too. Vitamin D actually strengthens the cell's defenses against viral attack by blocking viral replication. And vitamin D specifically targets the pro-inflammatory cytokines responsible for lung damage in pneumonia. And did I mention: it has antioxidant powers, too. [1]

One of the ways viruses attack cells is by breaking down the barriers and junctions between the cells. Vitamin D strengthens those barriers to keep the virus from invading the cells. [2]

Vitamin D strengthens the cell's inborn ability to fight off a broad spectrum of bacteria, fungi, and viruses by stimulating the cell's defensive proteins to, in effect, turn the tables on the invaders by attacking the microbe's own cell membranes and neutralizing the invader's toxins. [3]

. . .

Vitamin D And Dengue Virus

Vitamin D's anti-viral abilities have been well-tested. In one study, supplements of 1000 or 4000 IU were given to 20 healthy people for 10 days, then their blood samples were exposed to the dengue virus, which in some ways produces an illness that seems similar to COVID-19. The blood of people who received 4000 IU per day was much more resistant to the virus. Inflammatory cytokines were reduced and anti-inflammatory cytokines were increased. [4]

This beneficial modulation of cytokines is a common occurrence in vitamin D studies. That sentence makes it sound simple, but it's actually a complex cascade of effects on several vital elements of the immune system and a multitude of different cells, each with specific defensive purposes. [5] Vitamin D, much like garlic, is a conductor who not only modulates an array of instruments, but who also stimulates them to give their strongest performance.

The Anti-Viral Tag Team

In fact, vitamins D and C make up a kind of biochemical tag team. Vitamin D increases production of cellular antioxidants—which is turn "spare" or free vitamin C to perform its other protective duties.[6] A clinical study, in which vitamin D was added to a vitamin C supplement given to people with congestive heart failure, found that adding the vitamin D resulted in higher levels of an anti-inflammatory cytokine (IL-10). [7]

Vitamin D And Cytokines in Diabetes

Vitamin D status was measured in diabetic patients

with foot infections. The higher the vitamin D concentration in their blood, the fewer inflammatory cytokines. [8]

Vitamin D And ICU Patients on Ventilators

A Georgia study gave high dose vitamin D supplements to ICU patients on ventilators. Subjects were given either a placebo, 50,000 IU, or 100,000 IU daily for 5 consecutive days. The mean length of hospital stay was 36 days for the unsupplemented, 25 days for the 50,000 IU patients, and 18 days for the 100,000 IU patients. [9] A similar study of ICU patients on ventilators found that the higher daily dose, 100,000 IU for 5 days, increased the blood's ability to deliver oxygen to the cells. [10]

Vitamin D — A Seasonal Thing?

There is a lot of research around the theory that vitamin D's effects on the immune system can be demonstrated through the effects of the seasons on sunlight and vitamin D availability. I'll sum it up: Vitamin D levels are lower in winter because people are less exposed to the sun and their bodies can't manufacture as much of the vitamin. Therefore, higher incidence of respiratory infections in winter proves that vitamin D status determines our resistance to colds, flu, and pneumonia. In fact, there are scientists proposing that there are more serious COVID-19 infections in northern latitude countries because average vitamin D status is lower than in southern latitudes. [11] [12] [13] [14] [15] [16]

. . .

Vitamin D Blood Levels Make A Difference In Flu — And COVID-19

One study made the case by comparing actual vitamin D blood levels against flu infections: In 2009 researchers in Connecticut measured the blood levels of vitamin D in 198 healthy people over the course of flu season. They found that the people whose blood levels were greater than 38 ng/mL had *fewer than half* as many cases of acute respiratory infections as people whose levels were lower than 38 ng/mL. Of the higher levels group, only 17% percent came down with infections, whereas 45 percent of the lower blood level group did. [17]

Another study compared the vitamin D status of COVID-19 patients with the severity of their disease and the clinical outcome. They discovered that blood levels of vitamin D were highest in those with a mild cases and lowest in those with severe cases. Among the patients with the highest levels of vitamin D in their blood, more than 85 percent of the cases were mild. Among the patients who had insufficient or deficient levels, only about 2 percent of the cases were mild. [18]

Prevailing Scientific Opinion: Deficiency seriously weakens the immune system. Adequate intake supports healthy immunity. New research suggests a possible link to viral infection outcomes.

VITAMIN E

VITAMIN E DEFICIENCY IMPAIRS THE IMMUNE SYSTEM.
[1]Scientific evidence is accumulating that suggests the current recommended dietary levels of vitamin E might not be adequate to meet human needs at different life stages—in particular the immune system of elderly people. [2]

Animal studies have demonstrated that supplementing diets with extra vitamin E reduces inflammation and strengthens the immune system of older animals. And the results were reproduced in human studies as well. Healthy individuals 60 or older taking 800 mg per day (approx 1200 IU) saw their inflammation markers decrease and their immune strength increase.

When the same researchers tested other doses of vitamin E, they found that 200 mg (300 IU) had a stronger influence on immune strength than 0, 60, or 800 mg. Scientists believe vitamin E maintains the integrity of the cells fighting off the infection and preserves their ability to function as they age. [3]

. . .

Infection Fighter

Animal tests have demonstrated that vitamin E supplements protect from influenza infection in young and old animals—but more powerfully in older ones. Biochemically, vitamin E appears to increase infection-fighting cytokines when they're needed and inhibit inflammation when that's called for. [4]

A study looking back at the nutritional status and health of people over 60 found that blood levels of vitamin E were significantly lower the more prior infections they experienced. Another study demonstrated that healthy elderly people taking vitamin E supplements reported a lower incidence of infections. A similar study, of nursing home residents over 65, found that those receiving vitamin E supplements (300 IU per day) for one year had lower incidence of upper respiratory infections and colds compared to those who took placebo. [5]

We usually expect vitamin supplements to help protect us against the effects of unhealthy habits—like smoking. Apparently, this isn't the case with vitamin E. Studies comparing the effect of vitamin E supplementation on smokers and nonsmokers have found that while supplementation can reduce the respiratory infection and pneumonia rate for nonsmokers, for smokers it can actually increase the risk. [6] [7]

Vitamin E Reduces Cytokines

Vitamin E suppresses oxidation and cytokine inflammation that are believed to cause osteoporosis. Vitamin E not only neutralizes free radicals but also inhibits inflammation-promoting COX-2 enzyme. Smoking elevates pro-inflammatory cytokines, but vitamin E—particularly tocotrienol—blocks that elevation. Vitamin E also lowers levels of cytokines that weaken the bones. [8]

Vitamin E can also reduce cytokines generated during high-intensity interval training. In more than one study, animals given vitamin E reduced their levels of inflammatory cytokines compared to animals who were not supplemented. [9]

Exercise at high altitudes can stress the body in ways that the same exercise at sea level will not. Vitamin E protects red blood cells from free radical damage that occurs at high altitudes and maintains their ability to carry and deliver oxygen. [10]

Cancer patients undergoing therapy experience weakening of the immune system and high levels of chronic inflammation. A study in which cancer patients received supplements of approximately 1100 IU each day for two weeks found that their cytokines were brought more into balance, improving their immune function. [11]

Animal studies have demonstrated that vitamin E can improve immune function and suppress inflammatory cytokines, even in animals infected with HIV. [12] [13]

Prevailing Scientific Opinion: Deficiency weakens the immune system and promotes inflammation.

6

SELENIUM

USUALLY, SELENIUM IS DESCRIBED AS AN ANTIOXIDANT, but its role in the body is much more complex and powerful. Selenium is a major player in immunity and inflammation. Without adequate selenium, immunity hardly functions. Selenium is not only a structural element, but a regulatory one as well. The immune system needs selenium for its activation and regulation. It can be a factor in inflammation, viral immunity, autoimmune disease, sepsis, chronic autoimmune disorders, thyroid hormone metabolism, cardiovascular health, prevention of neurodegeneration, and cancer.[1]

One of the ways immune cells kill invaders is through an "oxidative burst." Selenium makes that burst bigger and more effective. This is one case where, at least in animal and test tube studies, extra selenium improves the immune system—by making the oxidative burst even stronger.[2]

In a controlled experiment, 22 adults received 50 or 100 mcg per day (That's *MICRO* grams) for 15 weeks. Their immunity to the polio virus was strengthened.

Another study found that supplements of 297 mcg per day increased antibodies to diptheria—but not influenza A or B. [3] Studies of selenium and other viral infections seem to suggest that in a deficiency state, the weakened immune system and increased oxidative stress allows the virus to mutate and become more virulent.[4]

Selenium supplementation has shown a protective effect against H1N1 influenza in animal studies. Only 25 percent of the deficient animals survived the infection. Only 41 percent of the animals fed "adequate" levels of selenium survived. But 75 percent of the animals fed extra selenium survived. [5]

Selenium Regulates Cytokines

Selenium does play a role in regulating cytokines. Measured in patients with liver cirrhosis, when selenium levels go down, inflammatory cytokines increase, and vice versa. [6] Women with gestational diabetes were given selenium to test its effect on inflammation. Selenium supplements of 200 mcg per day did reduce inflammatory cytokines. [7]

Deficiency in selenium during sepsis can bring about a deadly cycle in which a weakened immune system leaves the victim more vulnerable to what is called "critical illness stress-induced suppression," or CRISIS. As the CRISIS deepens, the immune system calls for more selenium and, not getting enough, weakens even further. [8]

Intervention with selenium supplementation has mitigated CRISIS in animal studies. [9] In humans, there have been a handful of studies but the results have not been encouraging. [10] [11]

Likewise with selenium treatment of a cytokine storm-like condition called SIRS, or Systemic Inflammatory Response Syndrome. Results have been mixed. In some studies, selenium treatment of critically ill patients with SIRS resulted in improvement and increased survival rates. But in others, it did not. [12]

Be Careful With Selenium

Selenium, like zinc, is absolutely necessary for a healthy immune system and does often require supplementation—but, also like zinc, can hurt you if you get too much. The catch-22 of selenium is that the difference between the amount that saves you and the amount that hurts you would not budge your spice scale. Small changes can make a big difference. [13]

Prevailing Scientific Opinion: Deficiency weakens the immune system and promotes inflammation, but supplementation must be done carefully to avoid toxic dose.

7

ZINC

I CAN SUM UP ZINC IN ONE SENTENCE: IT'S CRUCIAL TO A healthy immune system and helps block virus infections, but getting too much can be just as bad as getting too little.

About 30 percent of the world's population is estimated to be deficient in zinc—and that number does not exclude developed countries. In fact, studies have shown that about 30 percent of the elderly are zinc deficient and that it definitely affects their immune system, sense of taste, and wound healing. [1]

Zinc Supplements Boost Immunity

Zinc is absolutely necessary to an effective immune system, meaning that if you're deficient in zinc your immune system will be impaired, leaving you more vulnerable to infections. Because zinc also helps maintain immune balance, a deficiency can leave you more prone to inflammation. Zinc supplementation can usually correct a deficiency and re-invigorate the immune system. In developing countries, where zinc deficiency is prevalent in young children, supplementation has resulted in fewer cases of pneumonia. [2]

Studies in which the elderly were supplemented with zinc demonstrate improved immune strength. In one such study, 20 mg of zinc per day (with 100 mcg of selenium) resulted in a significant decrease in respiratory infections. Another study found 45 mg daily of zinc reduced the incidence of colds and fevers. A study of nursing home residents found that people with higher blood zinc levels had fewer cases of pneumonia, shorter duration of pneumonia, and less total use of antibiotics. [3]

Remember I said zinc is also important to balance in the immune system. Low zinc levels are not only associated with a weakened immune system, but also with inflammation and autoimmune disease. In human and animal studies, low zinc levels are linked to increased vulnerability to sepsis and fatality. [4]

Zinc And Sepsis

What about sepsis? Can zinc help prevent sepsis? There's evidence that it can be protective, in animal models and some human studies with newborns. [5] In adults, patients on ventilators have a much lower rate of pneumonia if they receive zinc supplements. [6] Another study found that patients with ARDS (acute respiratory distress syndrome) are more likely to have low zinc levels than non-ARDS patients. [7]

Researchers in one review concluded that a decade of scientific data established that zinc was essential to the body's resistance to sepsis and that experiments with humans as well as animals had demonstrated that it could be protective. [8]

But the evidence is not as clear as we'd like. It seems that not only does the human organism require zinc, but the invading pathogens often require it, too. Scientists believe that the body might sequester zinc from the blood and "hide" it in the liver during an infection to prevent the invader from using it, in addition to other immune-related functions. This is why you definitely do not want to flood your system with excess zinc. [9]

Zinc Lozenges

Lots of people swear by zinc lozenges. So does a noted virologist, apparently. Back in February, social media lit up with a letter written by the virologist to relatives advising them that zinc lozenges could block the coronavirus from infecting the throat and nasopharynx. When contacted by Snopes to confirm or deny, he confirmed—but hastened to add that zinc lozenges were not guaranteed protection against getting the virus. [10]

It turns out there is scientific evidence that zinc lozenges can help block coronavirus—not COVID-19, specifically, but a variant of coronavirus. A 2010 test tube study demonstrated that zinc blocks replication of coronavirus. [11] But there is at least one human clinical study, too.

Doctors at the Cleveland Clinic gave zinc lozenges or placebo to employees in the early stages of a cold. The people who received the actual zinc lozenges had significantly fewer days with symptoms—coughing, headache, hoarseness, nasal congestion, nasal drainage, and sore throat. The zinc group had more side effects, too: mostly nausea and bad-taste reactions. [12]

Zinc Helps—But Be Careful

Yes, zinc is necessary for a strong immune system. Yes, zinc supplements have been shown to improve immunity. Yes, zinc status is a factor in cytokine storm. But— also Yes—too much zinc can produce the same harmful effects as too little. When zinc concentrations become too high, immune system cells are damaged and inflammatory cytokines are produced. [13]

Zinc Has Been Called "The Essential Toxin" [14]

Zinc is toxic in excess amounts, but the likelihood of not getting enough is much greater than the chances you're getting too much. But how much IS too much? Well, the lethal dose is estimated to be 27 grams. You'd need to work pretty hard to get that much. Most zinc supplements are in the order of 10-30 *milligrams,* and taking much over 200 mg at one time will probably make you throw up. Nausea and vomiting have been reported in daily doses as low as 150 mg—a dose used in several supplementation studies without comparable side effects. That's not to say that a similar dose might not cause issues for you. Intake as low as 100 – 160 mg has caused lower HDL cholesterol (the "good cholesterol") and elevated levels of harmful LDL cholesterol. [15]

A study involving more than 46,000 men found that supplemental zinc in doses of up to 100 mg/day did not cause a higher risk of prostate cancer—but higher doses more than doubled the risk. [16]

In test tube experiments excess zinc induces pro-inflammatory cytokines while depressing beneficial T cells. In a human study, 83 healthy volunteers were given 110 mg of zinc three times per day. The treatment had a balancing effect on their immune system. The lymphocyte response was decreased in high responders and increased in low responders. [17]

Prevailing Scientific Opinion: Deficiency weakens the immune system and promotes inflammation, but supplementation must be done carefully to avoid toxic dose.

OTHER NUTRITIONAL SUPPLEMENTS

8

HESPERIDIN

Every time you drink orange juice you get some hesperidin. In fact, in many of the human studies I looked at, that's how the hesperidin was administered.

Hesperidin has antiviral power—at least in a test tube. Researchers who tested it concluded that hesperidin inhibits viral replication and stimulates cellular immunity. [1] In test tube and animal studies, hesperidin reduces levels of inflammatory cytokines and stabilizes biomembranes. [2]

Hesperidin's anti-inflammatory quality has been extensively demonstrated in animal studies. But the human clinical evidence mostly involves hesperidin's neuroprotective ability, which researchers believe is due to its anti-inflammatory effect. Hesperidin administered to healthy adults—via orange juice—improved their cognitive function and episodic memory. Unexpectedly, they also benefited from reduced diastolic blood pressure. [3]

In another study, healthy middle-aged men were given orange juice with extra hesperidin or a placebo drink.

Their cognitive functions and reflexes were significantly improved.[4]

Prevailing Scientific Opinion: No requirement established. Some evidence of benefit to the immune system but not as much research overall as for vitamins and some other nutrients.

9

QUERCETIN

QUERCETIN IS A FLAVONOID WITH A BROAD AND POWERFUL array of effects on the body. Quercetin strengthens the immune system and reduces inflammation on many fronts. It has demonstrated anti-viral, anti-microbial, anti-inflammatory, and anti-allergic potential in animal and human studies. [1]

Quercetin reduces inflammation before it can start by inhibiting inflammatory cytokines and enzymes. [2] An animal study found that quercetin pretty much inhibited the effects of overfeeding fructose. Blood glucose spikes were blocked, harmful LDL cholesterol and triglycerides were reduced, and good HDL cholesterol was increased.[3]

The anti-inflammatory, anti-convulsant, and anti-stress effects of quercetin were demonstrated in another animal study. Quercetin suppressed stress-induced inflammatory cytokine IL-1β, blocked fever seizures and increased levels of anti-inflammatory cytokine IL-10. [4]

. . .

Quercetin Works In People, Too—But Maybe Not The Way You Might Think?

In an experiment on healthy people, quercetin alone did not seem to have much anti-inflammatory effect. However, when combined with vitamin C, it seemed to boost vitamin C's antioxidant, anti-inflammatory effect. The researchers theorized that quercetin increased the bioavailability of vitamin C. [5]

Not So Fast!

But, actually, it turns out quercetin is more than just vitamin C's faithful sidekick.

One study gave 150 mg/day of quercetin to overweight *people* 25 – 65 years old and their systolic blood pressure came down in both normotensive and, even more, in hypertensive individuals.

Wait, there's more: their levels of inflammatory cytokine TNF-α also decreased. And so did oxidized LDL in their blood. [6]

They tested two different quercetin supplements against a placebo to treat symptoms of chronic inflammatory pelvic pain in prostatitis. The men who received the quercetin supplements for a month fared much better when symptoms and quality of life impact were measured. The men taking the placebo did not experience a significant fall in symptom score. But more than two-thirds of the men who received the quercetin alone (500 mg, twice daily) had at least a 25% improvement in symptoms. The men who received a supplement containing 500 mg quercetin with bromelain and papain added fared even better. At least 82% of them improved 25%. The mean NIH symptom score in the supplemented men fell from 21 to 13.1, a 33% drop. [7]

Quercetin supplements (1000 mg daily) or placebo were given to badminton players and after eight weeks the length of time they could play before becoming exhausted was measured. The players who received quercetin were able to play significantly longer (over 10%).[8]

A group of elite male cyclists were given either a vitamin supplement containing quercetin or one without for six weeks. Those who received the quercetin shaved more than three percent off their 30 km time trial and boosted their peak power. [9]

But what does this have to do the immune system and cytokines?

Quercetin—Anti-Inflammatory

Glad you asked. Another study with trained cyclists tested the effects of quercetin (1000 mg daily) alone or quercetin with EGCG against a placebo. After two weeks, their biomarkers for inflammation were measured before and after a strenuous series of rides. After three days of heavy exertion, both quercetin groups of cyclists had decreases in inflammatory cytokines and C-reactive protein, a significant marker for inflammation.

But in the cyclists who received the quercetin with EGCG, the anti-inflammatory effects were significantly more pronounced. C-reactive protein was reduced to half what it was in the placebo group, and inflammatory cytokine reduction was 39% greater. [10]

Another trial with cyclists—this time only 7 days of receiving a twice-daily quercetin supplement of 500 mg—found that their oxygen capacity increased modestly but their ride time until fatigue set in was boosted by more than 13 percent. [11]

In a test tube experiment quercetin was more effective than an anti-dermatitis drug cromalyn in calming inflammation. [12]

Quercetin supplements (500 mg/day) were given to women with rheumatoid arthritis. After 8 weeks, their inflammatory cytokines, morning pain and stiffness, and after-activity pain were significantly reduced compared to placebo. In fact, the number of patients with "active disease" significantly decreased. [13]

The ~~Cream~~ Anti-Inflammatory In Your Coffee

You've probably seen mainstream reports on the research that coffee drinking and caffeine reduces the risk of Alzheimer's Disease and Parkinson's Disease. Researchers delving a little deeper into that effect discovered that it was actually quercetin in coffee that was responsible for the protective effect. [14]

Research testing quercetin's effects on obesity have produced mixed results. In a 12-week study, supplements of 100 mg/day significantly reduced body fat percentage, particularly in the arm, and body mass index of overweight or obese people. Another similar study using 150 mg/day supplements found that quercetin decreased waist circumference and blood concentrations of triglycerides. A 12-week study used quercetin from extract of onion. People lost weight, and their body fat percentage and BMI were reduced. A similar study, however, found no effect. [15]

Prevailing Scientific Opinion: No requirement established. Abundant evidence of benefit to the immune system.

LUTEIN

LUTEIN IS A CAROTENOID ANTI-OXIDANT AND ANTI-inflammatory. There are test tube, animal, and human clinical studies in which it is found to protect the eye against macular degeneration and cataracts. [1]

In test tube studies, lutein blocks cytokines that cause inflammation. [2]

There are also studies in which lutein reduces inflammation in people with coronary artery disease. Researchers believe it can help reduce chronic inflammation. [3]

Lutein also appears to protect the immune system of diabetics from the oxidizing effects of high blood levels of glucose. [4]

Prevailing Scientific Opinion: No requirement established. Some evidence of benefit, but not enough clinical data with the immune system.

RESVERATROL

RESVERATROL IS A SUBSTANCE FOUND IN SEEDS AND SKIN of grapes and berries. As a defensive maneuver plants actually produce more resveratrol when they are stressed, infected, or threatened. Resveratrol has been studied and promoted for its effects as an antioxidant, antiaging, anti-inflammatory, anticancer, anti-allergy supplement. For the purposes of this book, we're concerned only with its antioxidant and anti-inflammatory properties. [1]

In one study, resveratrol was able to protect animals from a deadly sepsis-like lung inflammation. Whereas all of the animals given resveratrol survived, all who did not receive it died. Resveratrol reduced inflammatory cytokines in the animals' blood and lungs. [2]

Another study demonstrated that resveratrol inhibited replication of influenza virus in a test tube. The same researchers then gave resveratrol to animals infected with influenza and improved survival and decreased viral load. [3]

In a test tube study, resveratrol was superior to steroids

in reducing cytokines in human cells from COPD (chronic obstructive pulmonary disease). [4] In another test tube study with human cells, resveratrol decreased inflammatory cytokines in irritated fat-storing tissue. [5]

Prevailing Scientific Opinion: No requirement established. Some evidence of benefit to the immune system, but not enough clinical data.

12

NAC—N-ACETYL-L-CYSTEINE

NAC IS THE SUPPLEMENT FORM OF THE AMINO ACID cysteine.

NAC inhibits inflammation and oxidation, and has antimicrobial powers. It's been used therapeutically and supportively in cystic fibrosis, acetaminophen poisoning, chronic obstructive pulmonary disease, chronic bronchitis, detoxification, immunodeficiency virus infection, and mental disorders. [1] NAC reduces fatigue in healthy adults during muscle stimulation, resistive loading, handgrip exercises, and intense cycling. [2]

Although NAC is not an actual antibiotic, it breaks down biofilms in human pathogens. NAC has potent antibacterial effects against a wide range of bacteria that cause oral infections. [3]

NAC is such an effective anti-inflammatory that it is used to prevent toxicity in resinous materials used in dentistry. [4] NAC has been used to protect the oral mucous membranes against oxidation. [5]

. . .

NAC and Glutathione

NAC is a precursor of the glutathione, one of the body's main antioxidants. Because glutathione taken by mouth is broken down before actual glutathione can be absorbed, NAC is a better source.[6] NAC reversed inflammatory cytokine production and restored glutathione to pre-inflammation levels in animals. [7] NAC blocked the formation of inflammatory arthritis in another animal study. [8]

There is evidence that glutathione depletion contributes to acute respiratory distress syndrome (ARDS). In small clinical trials intravenous or inhaled NAC helped reduce mortality and morbidity in lung damage caused by smoke inhalation or ARDS. [9]

NAC The Antiviral, Anti-Inflammatory

In test tube experiments NAC blocks growth of the H5N1 virus and also prevents the virus from producing pro-inflammatory cytokines in lung cells. In their 2010 paper the researchers concluded NAC and similar antioxidants could be a beneficial treatment option in the event of a flu pandemic.[10]

NAC has been shown to improve patients conditions in chronic broncho-pulmonary diseases such as chronic bronchitis. Extended release tablets of 300 mg NAC given to people twice a day with chronic bronchitis resulted in significantly fewer sick days as well as fewer days when the chronic condition flared up. People not receiving the NAC had almost three times as many sick days. [11]

A review of several such studies found that a

prolonged course of oral NAC can prevent acute flare-ups of chronic bronchitis. [12]

NAC not only suppresses the immune system to reduce inflammation, but also stimulates the immune system to block infection. [13]

In HIV patients, oral NAC 600 mg for six months blocked progressive growth of the viral load and kept other immune factors stable. [14]

In a small group of patients with septic shock, infusions of NAC increased production of a protective and healing cytokine and shortened the ICU stay of survivors. [15]

Prevailing Scientific Opinion: No requirement established. Abundant evidence of benefit to the immune system.

13

PREBIOTICS

PREBIOTICS ARE NUTRIENTS THAT FEED THE microorganisms in your gut. As a result, short-chain fatty acids are released into the blood, where they can affect not only the GI tract but the entire body. And they do. In a good way.[1]

Prebiotics give rise to probiotics, so they share the benefits, which include strengthening—and balancing—the immune system to better fight off infections and avoid inflammation. Prebiotics improve the effectiveness of vaccines, while reducing the side effects. [2]

For Children And Adults

In infants, prebiotics reduce the incidence of respiratory infections, diarrhea, fever, febrile seizures, use of antibiotics, and duration of disease. Researchers noted that the immune system of the supplemented infants were stronger, with higher levels of a vital antibody.[3] [4]

In adults, 12 weeks supplementation with prebiotics

has been shown to reduce body weight, blood glucose, and insulin. In another study, prebiotics supplements (15 g/day) improved glycemic control in people with type 2 diabetes. Prebiotics lowered fasting glucose and triglycerides in people with impaired glucose tolerance. [5] Prebiotics reduced at least one symptom (pain, bloating, diarrhea, cramping, or flatulence) in 71 percent of lactose-intolerant people. [6]

Prebiotics reduce inflammation in people with chronic inflammatory diseases, such as Crohn's Disease. [7]

Prebiotics And Cytokines

Prebiotics have successfully reduced inflammatory cytokines in several clinical studies with people. In more than one, healthy people experienced an increase in anti-inflammatory cytokines and a decrease in pro-inflammatory cytokines when given prebiotics over a period of time. [8] [9] A study of women with type 2 diabetes found that prebiotics reduced their inflammatory cytokines and fasting glucose levels. [10]

Cocoa Is A Prebiotic

Researchers gave healthy volunteers a daily beverage with a high content of cocoa flavenols. After four weeks, they measured their gut microflora and found that the drink had increased growth of beneficial *Lactobacillus* and *Bifidobacterium* and significantly decreased levels of disease-causing *Clostridia.* Inflammatory markers and triglycerides were also lower. [11]

This might explain why test tube and animal studies

have found that chocolate has an anti-inflammatory effect.
[12]

Prevailing Scientific Opinion: No requirement established. Abundant evidence of benefit to the immune system.

14

PROBIOTICS

IF YOU EAT ACTIVE CULTURE YOGURT OR DRINK KEFIR, you're getting probiotics. Probiotics have been used to treat or prevent antibiotic-caused diarrhea, sepsis and colitis in premature infants, infant colic, periodontal disease, and ulcerative colitis. [1]

Wait. All of those diseases affect the gut—except one. It makes sense that enriching the intestinal environment with beneficial bacteria would help with gut diseases. But how did periodontal disease get in there?

That's why probiotics are in this book—because they don't just strengthen the immune system in the gut, but *all over the body.* Including the respiratory tract. [2] And not only do they stimulate the immune system but they also regulate it and induce anti-inflammatory cytokines to restore and maintain balance. They strengthen the immune system to clear out infections, while preventing an excessive response and inflammation. [3]

There are plenty of test tube and animal studies demonstrating that probiotics increase immune strength and decrease excessive immune inflammation. But what about controlled studies of their effects on people? We have those, too. In general, what they find is that healthy adults given probiotics for several weeks show stronger immune response. [4]

Shorter Colds, Less Pneumonia

In one study, nursing home residents supplemented for 13 weeks developed a stronger immune response to influenza virus after being vaccinated. A shorter period receiving supplements (seven weeks) had no effect.[5]

Other studies on elderly people found that probiotic-fermented milk reduced the duration of respiratory and gastrointestinal infections and resulted in fewer colds. Another study found a shorter duration of colds, but no change in the number. A later study of over 1000 people reproduced those results. Finally, people given probiotics had significantly fewer cases of pneumonia when they received probiotic-supplemented milk for 12 weeks. Measurements of their immune systems found them stronger, even for 12 weeks after supplements stopped. [6]

Probiotics strengthen the immune system of people of all ages to fight off respiratory infections. College students given probiotic supplements for 12 weeks got over their colds two days faster, missed fewer school days, and had fewer severe symptoms than students who did not. [7]

An Italian study found that adding probiotics to milk resulted in fewer cases of rhinitis, otitis, laryngitis, tracheitis, and, gastroenteritis.[8]

. . .

Probiotics And inflammation

When probiotics were given to volunteers with rheumatoid arthritis, their levels of a major inflammatory cytokine were reduced. Other studies have shown a reduction in inflammatory sepsis in probiotic-supplemented preterm infants and in adults following gastrointestinal surgery. [9] A study of children from age 3 months to 12 years critically ill with sepsis found that probiotic treatment for one week significantly reduced proinflammatory cytokines and increased anti-inflammatory cytokines. The children treated with probiotics tended to reduce their time in the ICU by more than two days. [10]

Prevailing Scientific Opinion: No requirement established. Abundant evidence of benefit to the immune system.

15

HONEY

MUCH AS I'D LIKE TO BE ABLE TO SAY THAT EATING ALL the honey you want is a good way to reduce inflammation... well, you know the rest of that sentence.

Actually, honey has been shown in animal studies to reduce inflammation. [1] This is a little surprising, because honey's oldest claim to DIY healthcare legitimacy is in wound healing, and it aids wound healing by stimulating *inflammatory* cytokines. [2]

But taken orally, honey appears to have the opposite effect. Half of the runners training intensely on treadmills were given 50 grams of honey a day for 10 weeks and their levels of cytokines were measured. After exercise, the runners who received honey had lower levels of inflammatory cytokines than the runners who did not. [3]

Scientists have demonstrated in test tube experiments that honey has prebiotic activity.[4] That, and the other research, is enough to make me feel a little better about putting honey on my oatmeal.

. . .

Prevailing Scientific Opinion: No requirement established. Some, but not much, evidence of benefit to the immune system.

16

OMEGA-3—FISH OIL

OMEGA-3 FATTY ACID FISH OIL SUPPLEMENTS ARE AMONG the oldest supplements to be used specifically to decrease inflammation. There are plenty of test tube and animal studies demonstrating success in reducing inflammation. And there are several studies in which omega-3 fish oil given to human volunteers with chronic inflammatory diseases reduced inflammation and inflammatory cytokines.

In this chapter, any reference to omega-3 oil refers to fish oil. That's because omega-3 fatty acids from fish oil (eicosapentaenoic acid (EPA) and docosahexaenoic acid (DHA) are over nine times more powerful anti-inflammatories than omega-3 oil from vegetable sources (alpha-linoleic acid (ALA). [1]

In several studies, omega-3 in doses averaging 3.5 grams per day given to rheumatoid arthritis patients have decreased the number of tender joints and swollen joints, reduced morning stiffness, improved grip strength, time to fatigue, physician's global assessment score, use of

NSAIDs and other drugs, and improved patient's assessment of pain. [2]

Too Much Omega-6 Oil In Our Diet

One of the problems with human studies of omega-3
supplementation is that omega-6 oils—supplied mostly by
vegetable oils and margarine—can counteract any anti-
inflammatory benefit of omega-3 oils. And, unfortunately,
the Western diet tends to be much higher in omega-6 oils
than omega-3. So it might take a higher dose to offset the
inflammatory effect of the omega-6 oils. [3] [4]

For example, high intake of vegetable oils has been
implicated in causing and/or perpetuating inflammatory
bowel disease. And, similarly to the effect in rheumatoid
arthritis, omega-3 fish oil supplements can reduce inflammation and prevent relapse. But to offset the effects of
vegetable oils, supplemental doses of fish oil averaged 4.5
grams per day. [5]

Omega-3 and Cytokine Storm

Because of the strong anti-inflammatory effects of
omega-3 oils, doctors have tested their ability to fight the
cytokine storm of acute respiratory distress syndrome
(ARDS)—with some success, but mostly mixed results. [6]

Early studies tended to use ALA (vegetable sources)
instead of DHA and EPA, so the results were not conclu-
sive. However, when researchers started using fish oil
omega-3s, the results became more promising. Neverthe-
less, even then they frequently mixed fish oil with an

omega-6 oil from seeds, which might have counteracted any positive effect. [7] [8] [9]

One study found that omega-3s resulted in a lower risk of mortality, shorter time needing a ventilator, and a shorter stay in the ICU. A study of early-stage sepsis found that patients who did not receive omega-3 supplementation more frequently went on to suffer organ failure and septic shock. Not all studies, however, have reached those conclusions. [10]

I think it's important to point out again that a diet that contains too much omega-6 oils (soybean oil, corn oil, cottonseed oil, sunflower oil) will counteract the benefits of omega-3 supplementation. [11]

Prevailing Scientific Opinion: No requirement established. Abundant evidence of benefit to the immune system.

17

ALA (ALPHA-LIPOIC-ACID)

IN TEST TUBE STUDIES, ALA SUPPRESSES INFLAMMATORY cytokines.[1]

There are many peer-reviewed reports and studies of ALA's effects on inflammation and cytokines. A high proportion of the studies test the effects in diabetic or pre-diabetic patients. Most—but not all—of the studies demonstrate that ALA can reduce inflammatory cytokines and other markers for inflammation. [2] [3] [4]

ALA has been tested and demonstrated promise as a treatment for diabetes, metabolic syndrome, high cholesterol, dementia, cancer, and other diseases. [5] It's not within the scope of this book to investigate those benefits. It does appear that scientists believe ALA could have some effectiveness in reducing inflammation.

Prevailing Scientific Opinion: No requirement established. Some evidence of benefit to the immune system.

HERBS

18

ANDROGRAPHIS PANICULATA (A. PANICULATA)

THIS HERB, ALSO KNOWN AS "THE KING OF BITTERS" IS A fixture of traditional herbal medicine in China, India, Thailand, and Malaysia, where it's widely used to treat sore throat, flu, and respiratory infections, among other things. It stimulates the immune system and dampens inflammation—our primary interest here. [1]

Animal and test tube studies have established the herb's antioxidant and anti-inflammatory ability, which it seems to exert by blocking a pivotal biochemical that activates inflammatory cytokines. Test tube studies have also established that the herb is antimicrobial, antibacterial, and antiviral against several viruses, including dengue, HIV, and Epstein-Barr. While strengthening the immune system it also appears to dampen inflammatory cytokines.[2]

A Real Lifesaver

In developing countries, where infectious diarrhea is

the principal cause of death in children under 5 years of age, *A. Paniculata* extract cured over 88 percent of cases. [3]

The herb appears to give symptomatic relief in upper respiratory infections and has been compared to acetaminophen. Controlled studies have found it can relieve sore throat, cough, fatigue, muscle soreness, fever, dry throat, sleeplessness, ear ache, and general malaise. Patients suffer fewer sick days and tend to declare themselves recovered sooner. [4] [5]

Side Effects

Women are typically advised to avoid it during pregnancy and men when they are trying to conceive.[6]

Prevailing Scientific Opinion: No requirement established. Some evidence of benefit to the immune system.

19

ASTRAGALUS

ASTRAGALUS HAS BEEN USED IN TRADITIONAL CHINESE medicine to treat respiratory infections and other diseases for thousands of years. [1]

Astragalus Can Set Off Cytokines

In one study, for example, healthy people were given supplements of astragalus. They quickly developed symptoms of fever, including elevated temperature, fatigue, headache, and malaise. Plus—their levels of circulating inflammatory cytokines went up. All the symptoms went away within a day. [2]

In an animal study, astragalus supplements were effective in reducing organ damage from sepsis—until the dose was elevated too high and the protective effect was reversed. [3]

Another animal study demonstrated a decidedly anti-inflammatory effect of astragalus supplements. Astragalus significantly decreased inflammation and its harmful effects in animals with colitis. [4]

There doesn't seem to be a wealth of clinical evidence that astragalus can be anti-inflammatory—but there is some: Astragalus given to children with asthma lowered inflammatory cytokines, increased anti-inflammatory cytokines, and improved their symptoms. [5]

Prevailing Scientific Opinion: No requirement established. Some evidence of benefit to the immune system.

CAT'S CLAW

CAT'S CLAW IS AN HERB FROM THE AMAZON RAIN FOREST used in Peruvian traditional medicine for digestive complains and arthritis. It has been established in test tube studies that the herb has antioxidant and anti-inflammatory ability. Cat's claw blocks cytokine production and reduces oxidative damage. [1]

In an animal study, cat's claw demonstrated an immunomodulatory effect, by shifting the cytokine balance more towards the anti-inflammatory cytokines. [2]

In humans, a cat's claw supplement was given to healthy men to test its effects on immunity after pneumonia vaccination. There were no toxic side effects, and cat's claw resulted in a stronger, longer lasting immune response after 5 months. [3]

Prevailing Scientific Opinion: No requirement established. Some evidence of benefit to the immune system.

CURCUMIN AND TURMERIC

THERE'S NO DOUBT THAT CURCUMIN IS A POWERFUL ANTI-inflammatory and antioxidant.

Several studies have found that curcumin supplements reduce muscle soreness and/or inflammation after intense exercise, and can help speed recovery. [1]

In a study of almost 400 people with osteoarthritis, curcumin (1500 mg/day) went up against ibuprofen (1200 mg/day) in a test of reducing pain and improving joint function. After 4 weeks, curcumin was working just as well as high-dose ibuprofen, except on the stiffness scale it was actually doing a little better. And the curcumin didn't cause nearly as much abdominal discomfort. [2]

Antiviral and Anti-Inflammatory

Test tube and animal studies show that curcumin suppresses inflammatory cytokines and also has antiviral activity against numerous viruses, including HIV, hepatitis, encephalitis, and H1N1. In animal studies, curcumin suppresses lung-damaging runaway inflammation. [3]

In 2015, doctors working with curcumin concluded that because it could apparently inhibit cytokines, it should be considered in treating people experiencing cytokine storm.[4]

The doctors also concluded that in order to achieve therapeutic blood concentrations of curcumin such treatments would need to be intravenous. Unfortunately, dietary curcumin is not absorbed very efficiently.[5] But there is one very simple way to improve absorption of curcumin: take it with piperine, the major active component of black pepper. Piperine can increase bioavailability of curcumin by 2000 percent. [6]

Prevailing Scientific Opinion: No requirement established. Abundant evidence of benefit to the immune system.

22

ECHINACEA

WHEN THE COVID-19 PANDEMIC FINALLY BEGAN TO crash into our American consciousness, there were reports that taking echinacea was a bad idea because it was reported to stimulate pro-inflammatory cytokines. When I started the research for this book, I soon discovered that the picture is more nuanced.

Echinacea—Antiviral And Anti-Inflammatory

There is a lot of scientific evidence that echinacea has antiviral *and* anti-inflammatory capability. The antiviral effect comes about precisely because echinacea stimulates infection-fighting cytokines that also happen to be pro-inflammatory. But echinacea also stimulates a cytokine (IL-10) that is *anti-inflammatory.* [1] The authors of one paper measuring that effect concluded that this effect could result in symptoms disappearing faster. [2]

A scientific peer-review of treatment and prevention trials found that eight out of nine early treatment trials reported generally positive results and three of the four prevention trials reported marginal benefits. [3]

In one of these studies, echinacea was given at the outset of symptoms and for a week afterwards. The blood of the people receiving echinacea had higher and more sustained levels of infection-fighting immune cells. [4]

Not all studies find that echinacea can fight off or reduce symptoms of respiratory infections. One study where echinacea was given for several weeks found only a small effect on risk of illness.[5]

Echinacea, The Anti-Inflammatory

In test tube studies, echinacea has been shown to stimulate *anti-inflammatory* cytokines. One study used a virus to stimulate cytokine release and then treated the cells with echinacea. The treatment succeeded in reversing the cytokine release and dampening inflammation.[6]

A similar study stimulated human bronchial cells with cold viruses. Echinacea not only reduced the inflammation but also directly blocked the growth of the virus.[7]

In a study where animals were infected with bacteria, echinacea activated the immune system's first defenses, which did include inflammatory, infection-fighting cytokines. Echinacea also reduced the number of bacteria. [8]

Prevailing Scientific Opinion: No requirement established. Abundant evidence of benefit to the immune system.

23

ELDERBERRY

Does elderberry increase cytokines or not?

In test tube experiments, elderberry extract has demonstrated effectiveness against at least 10 strains of influenza virus. In human studies it shortened flu symptoms to 3-4 days and seemed to produce more flu antibodies. However, when inflammatory cytokines were measured *in the drawn blood of healthy people* taking elderberry extract and compared to the effect of a known cytokine stimulant, the elderberry produced up to 45 times more inflammatory cytokines. [1]

Though it's a test tube experiment and not really an indication of what happens in the body, this could be a problem. In fact, there has been a lot of internet chatter warning people not to take elderberry, or to take it *until* the first sign of a serious infection.

I searched for published scientific evidence that elderberry exerted its antiviral effect without raising inflammatory cytokines or that it could reduce inflammatory cytokines. What I found were test tube or animal studies where elderberry extract exerted either a very mild anti-inflammatory effect [2], or a more or less neutral effect. [3] The only study I could find that measured inflammation markers in people given elderberry supplements found no significant change. [4] In the only study that had a clear inhibiting effect on inflammatory nitric oxide, specific cytokines were not measured. [5]

Prevailing Scientific Opinion: No requirement established. Some evidence of benefit to the immune system.

EUCALYPTUS

REMEMBER THAT GOOPY STUFF YOUR MOTHER RUBBED ON your chest when you had a cold or a cough? It contained eucalyptus. There actually are clinical studies in which people inhaled eucalyptus to relieve pain—and it worked! Not only did it relieve pain in patients after knee surgery, but it also lowered their blood pressure. [1]

Eucalyptus extract taken orally can have anti-inflammatory effects. Oral extract of eucalyptus was given to people with asthma (200 mg, three times per day for 12 weeks) and their lung function significantly improved. They also required fewer "rescue puffs" of medication than the control group, even though their regular asthma medication was reduced. [2]

Prevailing Scientific Opinion: No requirement established. Some evidence of benefit to the immune system.

GARLIC

GARLIC APPEARS TO BALANCE THE IMMUNE SYSTEM. WE tend to think of balance as implying stillness and, perhaps, weakness—and forget that balance can mean ferocious strength when it's called for and powerful calming when that is what's required.

There's nothing weak about garlic.

Garlic is one of the most powerful boosters of the immune system there is, and one of the most powerful anti-inflammatory agents as well. Garlic stimulates the immune system when you need it to be stimulated and calms it down when you need that. Garlic has scientifically proven ability as an antibacterial, antioxidant, antiparasitic, antiviral, anti-inflammatory, anti-allergenic agent. [1]

Garlic strengthens the immune system by stimulating and regulating a broad array of immune cells, including cytokines, lymphocytes, natural killer cells, and eosinophils. Garlic seems to act like the conductor of an orchestra, not only making sure all the different instru-ments play in harmony to give the best results, but stimulating them to give their most powerful performance. Those results have proved to be supportive in the treatment and prevention of a many diseases, including heart disease, gastric ulcers, obesity, metabolic syndrome, infections, and cancer, as well as a staggering array of microorganisms, including many viruses. [2] [3]

Garlic and Cytokines

In a test-tube experiment, garlic extract suppressed the production of inflammatory cytokines and raised levels of an anti-inflammatory cytokine. [4] Researchers then tested the ability of garlic to reduce inflammatory cytokines in postmenopausal women. They gave two garlic tablets a day to one group and a placebo to another. In the women who received the garlic tablets, inflammatory cytokines were cut almost in half (47%). [5]

Doctors gave 400 mg garlic extract twice a day to dialysis patients for eight weeks to test its ability to reduce serious cytokine inflammation. C-Reactive Protein, a biochemical marker used to measure inflammation, was reduced by over 70% in the patients who received garlic. [6]

Garlic, Colds and Flu

Over a three-month period doctors gave garlic tablets to 73 people and a placebo to 73 others and kept track of how many colds occurred in each group. In the garlic group there were 24 colds, compared to 65 in the placebo group. Garlic also shortened the average duration of colds by one day (4.63 vs 5.63). [7]

. . .

Fewer Sick Days

In another study of garlic and colds and flu, doctors found that garlic did not reduce the number of colds and flu infections but did dramatically reduce the humber of symptoms (by 21%), number of days where people performed sub optimally (by 61%) and number of school or work days missed (by 58%) due to illness. Garlic boosted natural killer cells and T lymphocytes. [8]

Garlic And Dengue Fever

Dengue is a mosquito-borne viral infection. World-wide, there are at least 100 million cases every year, and the WHO estimates there could be as many as 400 million. And though it's prevalent in tropical areas, there have been outbreaks in North America and Europe. Most cases are mild. But many progress into a severe, life-threatening flu-like illness. [9]

Sound familiar?

Inflammation plays a major role in the course of severe cases. Researchers believe oxidative stress to be the trigger for the inflammation. Because garlic reduces inflammation as well as oxidation, they tested garlic as a treatment. They found that garlic reduced the levels of three major inflammatory cytokines during the infection. [10]

Get Your Garlic Fresh

Even though some of the studies described in this chapter use garlic tablets or capsules, you might get more of the benefits if you use fresh raw garlic cloves.

Unfortunately, supplements might not be supplying

what you expect. A recent experiment found that most of the 24 garlic supplements tested did not deliver the stated dose of the active ingredient, allicin. The pills *contained* the stated amount, but because of excipients and lack of required natural factors, the supplements did not *release* more than 15% of their stated dose. [11]

Prevailing Scientific Opinion: No requirement established. Abundant evidence of benefit to the immune system.

26

GINGER

GINGER IS ONE OF THE MOST WIDELY CONSUMED FOODS IN the world. In some places it's just a condiment. In others, it's medicine. In traditional herbal medicine ginger is used to bring down fevers, shorten upper respiratory infections, calm nausea, bring down high blood pressure, soothe migraines, and relieve arthritis and other inflammatory diseases. [1]

For our purpose in this book, defense against viral infection and inflammatory cytokines, ginger is a triple threat. It inhibits oxidation, fights microbial infection, and reduces inflammation.[2]

Antioxidant

An animal experiment found that ginger's antioxidant power is comparable to vitamin C's. [3] Ginger works its antioxidant magic by raising levels of antioxidant enzymes and the body's onboard antioxidant, glutathione. [4]

· · ·

Antimicrobial

When administered before infection, fresh ginger blocked a deadly human respiratory virus from attaching to cells. Dried ginger did not have that preventive effect. [5]

Anti-Inflammatory

Ginger really comes into its own as an anti-inflammatory agent. Ginger suppresses inflammatory prostaglandins and blocks the synthesis of pro-inflammatory cytokines. It down-regulates inflammatory nitric oxide and COX-2, the enzyme responsible for inflammation and pain. [6]

Ginger given to diabetes patients lowered blood levels of cytokines responsible for chronic low-grade inflammation. [7] In a double-blind study, older people suffering from osteoarthritis were given 500 mg ginger supplements every day for three months—or a placebo. The levels of pro-inflammatory cytokines in their blood were measured at the beginning and end of the study. The folks who received the ginger supplements had significantly lower levels of inflammatory cytokines. [8]

Ginger And The Runners[9]

Running apparently stimulates a lot of cytokines, because researchers always seem to test anti-inflammatory agents on them. Maybe it's because so many researchers *are* runners? Anyway, two groups of well-trained runners were given either 500 mg of ginger three times a day —or a placebo. After six weeks of training and supplements, the runners who received the ginger supplements had significantly lower levels of inflammatory cytokines.

· · ·

Prevailing Scientific Opinion: No requirement established. Moderate amount of evidence of benefit to the immune system.

GINSENG

HERE'S THE PROBLEM WITH GINSENG: THERE ARE SEVERAL different varieties and each one has different effects. For example, some varieties are a sexual tonic, while others are more general in their effects. There's plenty of research on ginseng—and it does affect the immune system and inflammation. But it's all over the place in terms of what those effects are and which varieties have which effects,

For example, in one study, *Ginseng radix* stimulates inflammatory cytokines,[1] and in another, *Korean Red Ginseng,* has a stabilizing effect on cytokines in children receiving chemotherapy. [2]

In another study *aqueous* extract of *North American Ginseng* stimulated inflammatory cytokines while *alcohol* extract of the same variety suppressed inflammation. [3]

Prevailing Scientific Opinion: No requirement established. Some evidence of benefit to the immune system, but sorting out varieties can be difficult.

GOLDENSEAL AND BERBERINE

GOLDENSEAL IS WIDELY PROMOTED AS AN ANTIBIOTIC, anti-viral herb. I have seen and taken it bundled in an echinacea supplement. It turns out I was guilty of not doing my homework. There is no clinical evidence that goldenseal, or its active ingredient berberine, taken orally can fight a systemic infection or suppress inflammation. The evidence is all in test tube experiments. Goldenseal applied topically can effectively treat skin infections. But taken orally, no.

Prevailing Scientific Opinion: No requirement established. No clinical evidence of benefit to the immune system.

1

GREEN TEA—EGCG

THERE'S PLENTY OF EVIDENCE FROM TEST TUBE, ANIMAL, and human studies that green tea, or an extract of its most biologically active polyphenol, *epigallocatechin-3-gallate* (EGCG), strengthens the immune system and discourages inflammation. [1]

Dozens of test tube, or *in vitro*, experiments demonstrate that EGCG blocks cytokine-induced inflammation by actually "downregulating" the inflammatory cytokines themselves or preventing the white blood cells from following the cytokine's "orders" to attack friendly cells. Numerous animal studies confirm that the effect carries over to living creatures. [2] [3]

In animal experiments, green tea reduces the severity of autoimmune diseases like arthritis by increasing anti-inflammatory cytokines and inhibiting inflammatory cytokines.

Green Tea Can Help Ward Off Colds And Flu

Green tea strengthens the body's defenses against bacteria, viruses, fungi, and at least one parasite. Not only does green tea help fight the infections, it can help prevent them, too. Animal studies demonstrated that consumption of green tea can inhibit the actual transmission of bacteria and viruses. Studies with humans have had similar effects, resulting in fewer fever illness, fewer illnesses with cold or influenza symptoms, and fewer actual infections with Influenza A or B. [4]

Green Tea Is A Powerful Antioxidant

Green tea battles oxidation on several fronts. It blocks enzymes that cause inflammation and induces enzymes that neutralize it. Green tea can also scavenge free radicals and interfere with the molecular signaling that produces it. [5]

Green Tea And Sepsis

In a normal year, sepsis results in hundreds of thousands of deaths every year is the United States. There are doctors who believe green tea could help bring the death rate down. In animal studies, they discovered that giving EGCG during sepsis boosted survival from 53% of infected animals to 82%. The researchers discovered that EGCG actually reduces sepsis by blocking a substance that activates immune cells to produce more cytokines. [6] [7]

Another study found that EGCG protected both obese and lean animals from inflammation by reducing inflammatory cytokines and increasing anti-inflammatory cytokines.[8] EGCG also protected the liver of animals from damage normally caused by hepatitis. Inflammatory cytokines were almost completely suppressed. [9]

Green tea's anti-inflammatory abilities have also been demonstrated in humans. At the end of a six-month trial in which green tea was given to female smokers and inflammatory markers were compared to smokers not receiving green tea, the women who received green tea showed a significant decrease in biochemical markers for inflammatory cytokines. [10]

Prevailing Scientific Opinion: No requirement established. Abundant evidence of benefit to the immune system.

LICORICE

Licorice, or its active ingredient GLYCYRRHIZIN, has been studied as an anti-viral treatment, and intravenous glycyrrhizin has been used in Japan in the treatment of viral hepatitis. However, despite the fact that licorice is commonly thought of as candy, its use comes with some pretty hefty risks and side effects.[1]

Those side effects include high blood pressure, muscle weakness, decreased libido, erectile dysfunction, headache, congestive heart failure, and many more.[2]

In any case, the clinical use of glycyrrhizin as an antiviral treatment involves *intravenous* use. Taking safe doses of licorice orally does not raise blood levels high enough to do any good.[3]

Prevailing Scientific Opinion: No requirement established. Little or no evidence of benefit to the immune system.

LOMATIUM

THE STORY GOES THAT WHEN THE SPANISH FLU EPIDEMIC hit in 1917-1918, the Washoe Indians in Nevada seemed strangely immune to its effects. The white doctors seeing this miracle investigated and decided that what saved the Washoe from the Spanish Flu was the herb lomatium.

In test tube studies, lomatium does exhibit the ability to inhibit the growth of certain viruses and bacteria, including those that cause HIV and tuburculosis. But in a study in which seven different viruses were exposed to lomatium and other herbs, only one virus was inhibited by lomatium. [1]

Lomatium might not actually be antiviral at all. Herbalist Paul Bergner believes it's actually an expectorant, and the mucus production it stimulates is responsible for boosting host resistance to respiratory infections. The problem is that this effect can come with a nasty rash, literally, if the treatment is not administered correctly. [2]

Prevailing Scientific Opinion: I could find no studies in which lomatium was tested on animals or humans.

MILK THISTLE

SILYMARIN, AN EXTRACT FROM THE SEEDS OF THE MILK thistle plant, has been used for centuries in traditional medicine for treatment of liver diseases. [1] It's also reported to have antioxidant and anti-inflammatory powers. [2]

There are a lot of test tube and animal studies demonstrating various effects of milk thistle. In the test tube studies, milk thistle stimulates the immune system against infectious diseases, increases anti-inflammatory cytokines[3] and suppresses inflammatory cytokines. [4] [5] In animal studies, milk thistle decreases inflammation and liver damage. [6]

In a clinical study, milk thistle extract was given to dialysis patients with inflammatory anemia. The herb successfully inhibited inflammatory cytokines. [7]

Silymarin has been used to treat patients with cirrhosis of the liver, significantly improving the survival rate.[8] In hepatitis C patients, silymarin significantly decreased their viral load, although cytokine levels did not change. [9]

. . .

Prevailing Scientific Opinion: No requirement established. Some evidence of benefit to the immune system.

33

OLIVE LEAF

OLIVE LEAF HAS BEEN STUDIED AS AN ANTIOXIDANT, ANTI-inflammatory, anti-atherogenic, anti-cancer, anti-microbial, and, finally, anti-viral. All of these capabilities have been demonstrated in test tube and animal studies. [1]

But what about in people?

A group of 60 pre-hypertensive people were given either olive leaf or a placebo for six weeks. Olive leaf significantly lowered their blood pressure, total cholesterol, LDL cholesterol, triglycerides, and a single inflammatory cytokine. [2]

Another study gave olive leaf or placebo to healthy males and managed to reduce significant markers of inflammation. [3]

Olive leaf extract was given to cancer patients to test its ability to reduce inflammation from intensive chemotherapy. Olive leaf significantly reduced oral inflammation and levels of inflammatory cytokines in their saliva. [4]

In a nine-week study, high school athletes received olive leaf extract supplements and their incidence of colds and flu was measured. The number of colds and flu infections did not decrease, but their sick days were 28 percent fewer.[5]

Prevailing Scientific Opinion: No requirement established. Some evidence of benefit to the immune system.

34

OREGANO

A COMBINATION OF OREGANO AND THYME ESSENTIAL OILS were found to significantly decrease cytokine inflammation, reduce damage to inflamed tissue, and increase survival rates in lab animals with inflammatory disease. [1]

In test tube studies, oregano oil has been found to inhibit the major pro-inflammatory cytokines[2] and increase the production of anti-inflammatory cytokines. [3]

Oregano oil also has antimicrobial abilities. In a test tube study, it killed 11 antibiotic-resistant bacteria without producing any resistance to its effects. [4] Animal studies have shown it can kill fungal infections and substantially increase survival rates, sometimes even better than drugs. [5,6]

Oregano oil applied to 3rd degree burn wounds drastically reduced the bacterial load with no significant side effects. [7]

. . .

Prevailing Scientific Opinion: No requirement established. Little or no clinical evidence of benefit to the immune system.

OSHA

OSHA, or *LIGUSTICUM PORTERI*, IS AN HERB USED IN traditional Native American and Mexican medicine. It is reputed to have anti-viral effects. I was able to find a single test tube study in which the herb was able to protect immune cells from oxidation. [1] Other studies I found were irrelevant to immunity or inflammation.

Prevailing Scientific Opinion: No requirement established. Little or no evidence of benefit to the immune system.

PEPPERMINT

PEPPERMINT HAS DEMONSTRATED ANTIVIRAL, ANTI-inflammatory, and antioxidant ability in test tube studies. It's been tested against respiratory syncytial virus (a common virus causing cold-like symptoms) and found to decrease inflammatory cytokines, protect against oxidation, and inhibit replication of the virus. Other studies have found peppermint to have similar antiviral and anti-inflammatory powers against influenza A, herpes simplex, and HIV.[1]

I was not able to find any clinical studies of peppermint's ability to prevent or improve the symptoms of respiratory infections. The clinical studies that do exist are mostly about its use in irritable bowel syndrome and other diseases of the digestive tract.

Prevailing Scientific Opinion: No requirement established.Little or no clinical evidence of benefit to the immune system.

RED CLOVER

RED CLOVER HAS BEEN TESTED IN CLINICAL TRIALS AND shown to be effective in relieving the symptoms of menopause. In one study, women received 80 mg/day for 90 days, and then after a one-week washout period receiving no supplement, switched places with the controls receiving a placebo. The prior controls then received the supplement for 90 days. This is known as a cross-over study. Because neither the doctors nor the women knew who was getting what, it was also "double-blind." In the 53 women who completed the study, red clover significantly reduced their menopausal symptoms. Also, their total cholesterol, LDL cholesterol, and triglyceride levels also decreased. [1]

Another, similar, study found that red clover prevented loss of bone density. [2] A third study found that red clover significantly reduced frequency of hot flashes.[3]

These studies establish that red clover has anti-inflammatory ability, at least in menopause. But the studies did not measure cytokines, so we don't know if red clover can reduce cytokine inflammation. There are test tube studies in which red clover suppresses inflammatory cytokines and blocks the release of a pro-inflammatory mediator.[4]

Prevailing Scientific Opinion: No requirement established. Some evidence of benefit to the immune system.

38

ST JOHN'S WORT

MOST OF US THINK OF ST. JOHN'S WORT AS AN antidepressant. But there's actually a lot of scientific proof that it also has antiviral, antibacterial, anti-cancer, anti-tumor, and anti-inflammatory properties. In fact, its antidepressant effect could be due to its powerful dampening effect on inflammation. [1] [2]

In a test tube experiment, St. John's Wort not only reduced inflammatory cytokines but also protected the targeted cells from cytokine damage. [3] The herb, at least in part, appears to work its anti-inflammatory effect by acting on prostaglandins, which are major regulators of inflammation. [4]

The scientific literature as well as the popular media are filled with warnings about how St. John's Wort can interact and interfere with prescription drugs. I wonder if that's because the drug companies are afraid it will seriously reduce their profits from antidepressants, since the list seems longer than for any other herb. It could also be a tip-off that the herb has some really powerful effects. In any case, here is the list of drugs with which St. John's Wort potentially interacts:

Alprazolam (Xanax), any antidepressant, barbiturates, bupropion, chemotherapy drugs, immunosuppressive drugs, tacrolimus, cyclosporine, statins, contraceptives, cytochrome, dextromethorphan, digoxin, fexofenadine, ketamine, methadone, meperidine, non-nucleoside reverse transcriptase inhibitors, anti-HIV drugs, omeprazole, phenytoin, photosensitizing drugs, protease inhibitors, triptans (migraine drugs), voriconazole, and warfarin. [5]

Prevailing Scientific Opinion: No requirement established. Some evidence of benefit to the immune system.

ALSO BY DOMINICK BOSCO

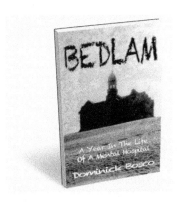

"Educational, uplifting, heartbreaking. What more could you want from a delicious read?" --S'Parks' 5-star Amazon review

"An eye-opening experience. A troubling book, difficult to put down...."—Library Journal

"By the time I reached the final chapter I found myself wishing there was more. I didn't want the story to have ended." — from the foreword by Katherine Broderick Anderson

ALSO BY DOMINICK BOSCO

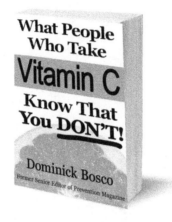

What do people who take vitamin C know that you don't? PLENTY!

The scientific facts about vitamin C and colds.

2 embarrassing situations where vitamin C can help you heal FASTER!

9 reasons why your cardiologist is taking vitamin C!

And much, much more!

ALSO BY DOMINICK BOSCO

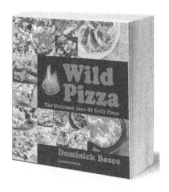

I just finished reading Wild Pizza and I'm starving! Not only are the recipes clever and fairly simple, they spark my culinary imagination. Chicken and capers? Fried green tomatoes? Chocolate chips? Yes, please! Bosco makes a case for cooking pizza on the grill — a novel addition to the summer outdoor cooking season. And his breezy style makes for a pleasant read.
—5-Star Amazon review

Awesome book! Great creative recipes in a useful and fun format…. A must have for the summer grilling season. —5-Star Amazon review

A NOTE ABOUT THE NOTES...

The endnotes for this book were originally intended to serve as links in an ebook. Since these links won't work in a printed book, you can download a pdf copy of the notes with working links from our website.

There is no charge and you will not need to enter an email address.

Copy this link in your browser and hit enter/return and you will go to a page where you can download the endnotes.

https://storyhillcreative.com/notes/

NOTES

1. Vitamin A

1. **VITAMIN A AS AN ANTI-INFECTIVE AGENT**
2. **Role of Vitamin A in the Immune System**
3. **Role of Vitamin A in the Immune System**
4. **Vitamin A as an anti-inflammatory agent**
5. **Role of Vitamin A in the Immune System**
6. **Vitamin A as an anti-inflammatory agent**
7. Vitamin A supplementation reduces the Th17-Treg – Related cytokines in obese and non-obese women
8. **Vitamin A as an anti-inflammatory agent**
9. **Vitamin A as an anti-inflammatory agent**
10. **Vitamin A as an anti-inflammatory agent**

2. B Vitamins

1. The effects of vitamin B on the immune/cytokine network and their involvement in depression
2. The effects of vitamin B on the immune/cytokine network and their involvement in depression
3. The effects of vitamin B on the immune/cytokine network and their involvement in depression
4. **HMGB1 Inhibition During Zymosan-Induced Inflammation: The Potential Therapeutic Action of Riboflavin**
5. The effects of vitamin B on the immune/cytokine network and their involvement in depression
6. **High dietary niacin intake is associated with decreased chromosome translocation frequency in airline pilots.**
7. **The long-term relationship between dietary pantothenic acid intake and C-reactive protein concentration in adults aged 40 years and older.**
8. The effects of vitamin B on the immune/cytokine network and their involvement in depression

9. Plasma Pyridoxal-5-Phosphate Is Inversely Associated with Systemic Markers of Inflammation in a Population of U.S. Adults

10. **Vitamin B6 supplementation improves pro-inflammatory responses in patients with rheumatoid arthritis**

11. The effects of vitamin B on the immune/cytokine network and their involvement in depression

12. **Folic acid supplementation improves cognitive function by reducing the levels of peripheral inflammatory cytokines in elderly Chinese subjects with MCI**

13. The effects of vitamin B on the immune/cytokine network and their involvement in depression

14. **Association of Vitamin B12 with Pro-Inflammatory Cytokines and Biochemical Markers Related to Cardiometabolic Risk in Saudi Subjects**

15. **Novel insight on the impact of choline-deficiency in sepsis**

16. **Inositol for respiratory distress syndrome in preterm infants**

17. Inositol and pulmonary function. Could myo-inositol treatment downregulate inflammation and cytokine release syndrome in SARS-CoV-2?

18. Biotin Deficiency Induces Th1- and Th17-MediatedProinflammatory Responses in Human CD4+T Lymphocytesvia Activation of the mTOR Signaling Pathway

19. **Biotin deficiency enhances the inflammatory response of human dendritic cells**

3. Vitamin C

1. New study identifies characteristics of patients with fatal COVID-19

2. **Clinical Features of 85 Fatal Cases of COVID-19 from Wuhan: A Retrospective Observational Study**

3. The Influence Of Vitamin C On Eosinophil Response To Acute Alcohol Intoxication In Rats

4. ISRN Vet Sci. 2011; 2011: 749753

5. Extra Dose of Vitamin C Based on a Daily Supplementation Shortens the Common Cold: A Meta-Analysis of 9 Randomized Controlled Trials

6. The effectiveness of vitamin C in preventing and relieving the symptoms of virus-induced respiratory infections.

7. Vitamin C Is an Essential Factor on the Anti-viral Immune

Responses through the Production of Interferon-α/β at the Initial Stage of Influenza A Virus (H3N2) Infection

8. Effects of L-ascorbic acid on the production of pro-inflammatory and anti-inflammatory cytokines in C57BL/6 mouse splenocytes

9. Effects of Vitamin C or E on the Pro-inflammatory Cytokines, Heat Shock Protein 70 and Antioxidant Status in Broiler Chicks under Summer Conditions

10. **Hydrocortisone, Vitamin C, and Thiamine for the Treatment of Severe Sepsis and Septic Shock: A Retrospective Before-After Study.**

11. **Phase I safety trial of intravenous ascorbic acid in patients with severe sepsis.**

12. **Influence of Vitamin C Supplementation on Cytokine Changes Following an Ultramarathon**

13. Vitamin C for preventing and treating pneumonia.

14. Vitamin C Mitigates Oxidative Stress and Tumor Necrosis Factor-Alpha in Severe Community-Acquired Pneumonia and LPS-Induced Macrophages

15. Vitamin C pharmacokinetics of plain and slow release formulations in smokers.

4. Vitamin D

1. **Evidence that Vitamin D Supplementation Could Reduce Risk of Influenza and COVID-19 Infections and Deaths**

2. **Evidence that Vitamin D Supplementation Could Reduce Risk of Influenza and COVID-19 Infections and Deaths**

3. **Evidence that Vitamin D Supplementation Could Reduce Risk of Influenza and COVID-19 Infections and Deaths**

4. Effect of high doses of vitamin D supplementation on dengue virus replication, Toll-like receptor expression, and cytokine profiles on dendritic cells

5. **Evidence that Vitamin D Supplementation Could Reduce Risk of Influenza and COVID-19 Infections and Deaths**

6. **Evidence that Vitamin D Supplementation Could Reduce Risk of Influenza and COVID-19 Infections and Deaths**

7. **Vitamin D supplementation improves cytokine profiles in patients with congestive heart failure: a double-blind, randomized, placebo-controlled trial.**

8. **Vitamin D deficiency is associated with inflammatory cytokine concentrations in patients with diabetic foot infection**

9. **High dose vitamin D administration in ventilated intensive care unit patients: A pilot double blind randomized controlled trial**
10. **High-Dose Vitamin D3 Administration Is Associated With Increases in Hemoglobin Concentrations in Mechanically Ventilated Critically Ill Adults: A Pilot Double-Blind, Randomized, Placebo-Controlled Trial**
11. Letter: Covid-19, and vitamin D
12. Do Latitude and Ozone Concentration Predict COVID-2019 Cases in 34 Countries?
13. **Vitamin D Supplementation Could Reduce the Risk of Type A Influenza Infection and Subsequent Pneumonia**
14. **Evidence that Vitamin D Supplementation Could Reduce Risk of Influenza and COVID-19 Infections and Deaths**
15. **Serum 25-Hydroxyvitamin D and the Incidence of Acute Viral Respiratory Tract Infections in Healthy Adults**
16. **Vitamin D and Influenza—Prevention or Therapy?**
17. **Serum 25-Hydroxyvitamin D and the Incidence of Acute Viral Respiratory Tract Infections in Healthy Adults**
18. Vitamin D Supplementation Could Possibly Improve Clinical Outcomes of Patients Infected with Coronavirus-2019

5. Vitamin E

1. Nutritional Modulation of Immune Function: Analysis of Evidence, Mechanisms, and Clinical Relevance
2. Nutritional Modulation of Immune Function: Analysis of Evidence, Mechanisms, and Clinical Relevance
3. Nutritional Modulation of Immune Function: Analysis of Evidence, Mechanisms, and Clinical Relevance
4. Nutritional Modulation of Immune Function: Analysis of Evidence, Mechanisms, and Clinical Relevance
5. Nutritional Modulation of Immune Function: Analysis of Evidence, Mechanisms, and Clinical Relevance
6. **Subgroup analysis of large trials can guide further research: a case study of vitamin E and pneumonia**
7. **The effect of vitamin E on common cold incidence is modified by age, smoking and residential neighborhood**
8. **The Anti-Inflammatory Role of Vitamin E in Prevention of Osteoporosis**
9. **Effect of vitamin E succinate on inflammatory cytokines induced by high-intensity interval training**

10. Effect of vitamin E supplementation on hypoxia-induced oxidative damage in male albino rats.

11. A Short-Term Dietary Supplementation of High Doses of Vitamin E Increases T Helper 1 Cytokine Production in Patients with Advanced Colorectal Cancer

12. Supplementing alpha-tocopherol (vitamin E) and vitamin D3 in high fat diet decrease IL-6 production in murine epididymal adipose tissue and 3T3-L1 adipocytes following LPS stimulation

13. Vitamin E supplementation modulates cytokine production by thymocytes during murine AIDS

6. Selenium

1. The Role of Selenium in Inflammation and Immunity: From Molecular Mechanisms to Therapeutic Opportunities

2. The Role of Selenium in Inflammation and Immunity: From Molecular Mechanisms to Therapeutic Opportunities

3. The Role of Selenium in Inflammation and Immunity: From Molecular Mechanisms to Therapeutic Opportunities

4. The Role of Selenium in Inflammation and Immunity: From Molecular Mechanisms to Therapeutic Opportunities

5. The Role of Selenium in Inflammation and Immunity: From Molecular Mechanisms to Therapeutic Opportunities

6. Association between Serum Selenium Concentrations and Levels of Proinflammatory and Profibrotic Cytokines—Interleukin-6 and Growth Differentiation Factor-15, in Patients with Alcoholic Liver Cirrhosis

7. Effects of Selenium Supplementation on Gene Expression Levels of Inflammatory Cytokines and Vascular Endothelial Growth Factor in Patients with Gestational Diabetes

8. The Role of Selenium in Inflammation and Immunity: From Molecular Mechanisms to Therapeutic Opportunities

9. The Role of Selenium in Inflammation and Immunity: From Molecular Mechanisms to Therapeutic Opportunities

10. Pharmaconutrition With Selenium in Critically Ill Patients

11. High-dose intravenous selenium does not improve clinical outcomes in the critically ill: a systematic review and meta-analysis

12. The Role of Selenium in Inflammation and Immunity: From Molecular Mechanisms to Therapeutic Opportunities

13. **The Role of Selenium in Inflammation and Immunity: From Molecular Mechanisms to Therapeutic Opportunities**

7. Zinc

1. Nutritional Modulation of Immune Function: Analysis of Evidence, Mechanisms, and Clinical Relevance
2. Nutritional Modulation of Immune Function: Analysis of Evidence, Mechanisms, and Clinical Relevance
3. Nutritional Modulation of Immune Function: Analysis of Evidence, Mechanisms, and Clinical Relevance
4. Nutritional Modulation of Immune Function: Analysis of Evidence, Mechanisms, and Clinical Relevance
5. Nutritional Modulation of Immune Function: Analysis of Evidence, Mechanisms, and Clinical Relevance
6. Zinc Supplementation in Adult Mechanically Ventilated Trauma Patients is Associated with Decreased Occurrence of Ventilator-associated Pneumonia: A Secondary Analysis of a Prospective, Observational Study
7. ZINC DEFICIENCY PRIMES THE LUNG FOR VENTILATOR INDUCED LUNG INJURY
8. **Souffriau J, Libert C. Mechanistic insights into the protective impact of zinc on sepsis. Cytokine Growth Factor Rev. (2018) 39:92–101. 10.1016/j.cytogfr.2017.12.002**
9. Nutritional Modulation of Immune Function: Analysis of Evidence, Mechanisms, and Clinical Relevance
10. **Did a Noted Pathologist Write This Viral Coronavirus Advice Letter?**
11. **Zn Inhibits Coronavirus and Arterivirus RNA Polymerase Activity In Vitro and Zinc Ionophores Block the Replication of These Viruses in Cell Culture**
12. **Zinc Gluconate Lozenges for Treating the Common Cold: A Randomized, Double-Blind, Placebo-Controlled Study**
13. **Zinc-altered immune function**
14. **The Essential Toxin: Impact of Zinc on Human Health**
15. **The Essential Toxin: Impact of Zinc on Human Health**
16. **The Essential Toxin: Impact of Zinc on Human Health**
17. **The Essential Toxin: Impact of Zinc on Human Health**

8. Hesperidin

1. A dual character of flavonoids in influenza A virus replication and spread through modulating cell-autonomous immunity by MAPK signaling pathways
2. Hesperidin as a Neuroprotective Agent: A Review of Animal and Clinical Evidence
3. Hesperidin as a Neuroprotective Agent: A Review of Animal and Clinical Evidence
4. Hesperidin as a Neuroprotective Agent: A Review of Animal and Clinical Evidence

9. Quercetin

1. The Role of Quercetin, Flavonols and Flavones in Modulating Inflammatory Cell Function
2. Therapeutic effects of quercetin on early inflammation in hypertriglyceridemia-related acute pancreatitis and its mechanism
3. Flaxseed and quercetin improve anti-inflammatory cytokine level and insulin sensitivity in animal model of metabolic syndrome, the fructose-fed rats
4. The Effect of Quercetin on Pro- and Anti-Inflammatory Cytokines in a Prenatally Stressed Rat Model of Febrile Seizures
5. The effect of quercetin supplementation on selected markers of inflammation and oxidative stress
6. Quercetin reduces systolic blood pressure and plasma oxidised low-density lipoprotein concentrations in overweight subjects with a high-cardiovascular disease risk phenotype: a double-blinded, placebo-controlled cross-over study
7. QUERCETIN IN MEN WITH CATEGORY III CHRONICPRO-STATITIS: A PRELIMINARY PROSPECTIVE, DOUBLE-BLIND, PLACEBO-CONTROLLED TRIAL
8. Effect of Eight Weeks of Quercetin Supplementation on Exercise Performance, Muscle Damage and Body Muscle in Male Badminton Players
9. Dietary antioxidant supplementation combined with quercetin improves cycling time trial performance.

10. Effects of quercetin and EGCG on mitochondrial biogenesis and immunity.
11. The dietary flavonoid quercetin increases VO(2max) and endurance capacity.
12. Quercetin is more effective than cromolyn in blocking human mast cell cytokine release and inhibits contact dermatitis and photosensitivity in humans.
13. The Effect of Quercetin on Inflammatory Factors and Clinical Symptoms in Women with Rheumatoid Arthritis: A Double-Blind, Randomized Controlled Trial.
14. Quercetin, not caffeine, is a major neuroprotective component in coffee.
15. The Beneficial Effects of Quercetin, Curcumin, and Resveratrol in Obesity

10. Lutein

1. The Role of Lutein in Eye-Related Disease
2. Abstract 580: Lutein Reduces Inflammation in Patients With Coronary Artery Disease by Suppressing Cytokine and Matrix Metalloproteinase-9 Secretion From Peripheral Blood Mononuclear Cells
3. Lutein exerts anti-inflammatory effects in patients with coronary artery disease.
4. Lutein prevents the effect of high glucose levels on immune system cells in vivo and in vitro.

11. Resveratrol

1. Properties of Resveratrol: *In Vitro* and *In Vivo* Studies about Metabolism, Bioavailability, and Biological Effects in Animal Models and Humans
2. Resveratrol protects mice against SEB−induced acute lung injury and mortality by miR−193a modulation that targets TGF−β signalling
3. Inhibition of Influenza A Virus Replication by Resveratrol
4. Resveratrol is superior to dexamethasone in suppressing cytokine release from human airway smooth muscle cells exposed to lipoteichoic acid in COPD
5. Obesity and inflammation: reduced cytokine expression due to

resveratrol in a human *in vitro* model of inflamed adipose tissue

12. NAC—N-acetyl-l-cysteine

1. Biological Activities and Potential Oral Applications of N-Acetylcysteine: Progress and Prospects
2. Free radicals and muscle fatigue: Of ROS, canaries, and the IOC.
3. Biological Activities and Potential Oral Applications of N-Acetylcysteine: Progress and Prospects
4. Biological Activities and Potential Oral Applications of N-Acetylcysteine: Progress and Prospects
5. Biological Activities and Potential Oral Applications of N-Acetylcysteine: Progress and Prospects
6. Biological Activities and Potential Oral Applications of N-Acetylcysteine: Progress and Prospects
7. N-acetylcysteine expresses powerful anti-inflammatory and antioxidant activities resulting in complete improvement of acetic acid-induced colitis in rats.
8. Effects of bucillamine and N-acetyl-l-cysteine on cytokine production and collagen-induced arthritis (CIA)
9. Emerging Therapies for the Prevention of Acute Respiratory Distress Syndrome
10. N-acetyl-l-cysteine (NAC) inhibits virus replication and expression of pro-inflammatory molecules in A549 cells infected with highly pathogenic H5N1 influenza A virus
11. Reduction in days of illness after long-term treatment with N-acetylcysteine controlled-release tablets in patients with chronic bronchitis.
12. Efficacy of oral long-term N-acetylcysteine in chronic bronchopulmonary disease: a meta-analysis of published double-blind, placebo-controlled clinical trials.
13. Long-Time Treatment by Low-Dose *N*-Acetyl-L-Cysteine Enhances Proinflammatory Cytokine Expressions in LPS-Stimulated Macrophages
14. The effect of N-acetylcysteine supplementation upon viral load, CD4, CD8, total lymphocyte count and hematocrit in individuals undergoing antiretroviral treatment.
15. Does N-Acetyl-L-Cysteine Influence Cytokine Response During Early Human Septic Shock?

13. Prebiotics

1. Prebiotics: Definition, Types, Sources, Mechanisms, and Clinical Applications
2. Prebiotics: Definition, Types, Sources, Mechanisms, and Clinical Applications
3. Effects of Probiotics, Prebiotics, and Synbiotics on Human Health
4. Prebiotics: Definition, Types, Sources, Mechanisms, and Clinical Applications
5. Effects of Probiotics, Prebiotics, and Synbiotics on Human Health
6. Effects of Probiotics, Prebiotics, and Synbiotics on Human Health
7. Effects of Probiotics, Prebiotics, and Synbiotics on Human Health
8. The Role of Probiotics and Prebiotics in the Prevention and Treatment of Obesity
9. Modulation of the fecal microflora profile and immune function by a novel trans-galactooligosaccharide mixture (B-GOS) in healthy elderly volunteers.
10. Oligofructose-enriched inulin improves some inflammatory markers and metabolic endotoxemia in women with type 2 diabetes mellitus: a randomized controlled clinical trial.
11. Prebiotic evaluation of cocoa-derived flavanols in healthy humans by using a randomized, controlled, double-blind, crossover intervention study.
12. The effects of cocoa on the immune system

14. Probiotics

1. Probiotics: What You Need To Know
2. Probiotics: What You Need To Know
3. Probiotics: What You Need To Know
4. Probiotics: What You Need To Know
5. Probiotics: What You Need To Know
6. Probiotics: What You Need To Know
7. Effect of Lactobacillus rhamnosus LGG® and Bifidobacterium animalis ssp. lactis BB-12® on health-related quality of

life in college students affected by upper respiratory infections.

8. Probiotics in Autoimmune and Inflammatory Disorders
9. Probiotics in Autoimmune and Inflammatory Disorders
10. Evaluation of Effect of Probiotics on Cytokine Levels in Critically Ill Children With Severe Sepsis: A Double-Blind, Placebo-Controlled Trial.

15. Honey

1. Immune response in rats following administration of honey with sulfonamides residues
2. Honey stimulates inflammatory cytokine production from monocytes.
3. Oral supplementation of natural honey and levels of inflammatory and anti- inflammatory plasma cytokines during 10-week of intensive treadmill training in endurance-trained athletes.
4. In vitro investigation into the potential prebiotic activity of honey oligosaccharides.

16. Omega-3—Fish Oil

1. n−3 Polyunsaturated fatty acids, inflammation, and inflammatory diseases
2. n−3 Polyunsaturated fatty acids, inflammation, and inflammatory diseases
3. n−3 Polyunsaturated fatty acids, inflammation, and inflammatory diseases
4. Importance of maintaining a low omega–6/omega–3 ratio for reducing inflammation
5. n−3 Polyunsaturated fatty acids, inflammation, and inflammatory diseases
6. The Role of Omega-3 Polyunsaturated Fatty Acids in the Treatment of Patients with Acute Respiratory Distress Syndrome: A Clinical Review
7. The Role of Omega-3 Polyunsaturated Fatty Acids in the Treatment of Patients with Acute Respiratory Distress Syndrome: A Clinical Review
8. Importance of maintaining a low omega–6/omega–3 ratio for reducing inflammation

9. Omega-6 vegetable oils as a driver of coronary heart disease: the oxidized linoleic acid hypothesis
10. **The Role of Omega-3 Polyunsaturated Fatty Acids in the Treatment of Patients with Acute Respiratory Distress Syndrome: A Clinical Review**
11. **n−3 Polyunsaturated fatty acids, inflammation, and inflammatory diseases**

17. ALA (alpha-lipoic-acid)

1. **Alpha-Lipoic Acid Suppresses Extracellular Histone-Induced Release of the Inflammatory Mediator Tumor Necrosis Factor-α by Macrophages**
2. **Effects of alpha-lipoic acid supplementation on C-reactive protein level: A systematic review and meta-analysis of randomized controlled clinical trials**
3. **The effects of alpha-lipoic acid supplementation on inflammatory markers among patients with metabolic syndrome and related disorders: a systematic review and meta-analysis of randomized controlled trials**
4. **Alpha-lipoic acid (ALA) supplementation effect on glycemic and inflammatory biomarkers: A Systematic Review and meta-analysis**
5. **Insights on the Use of α-Lipoic Acid for Therapeutic Purposes**

18. Andrographis Paniculata (A. Paniculata)

1. **Experimental and Clinical Pharmacology of *Andrographis paniculata* and Its Major Bioactive Phytoconstituent Andrographolide**
2. **Experimental and Clinical Pharmacology of *Andrographis paniculata* and Its Major Bioactive Phytoconstituent Andrographolide**
3. **Experimental and Clinical Pharmacology of *Andrographis paniculata* and Its Major Bioactive Phytoconstituent Andrographolide**
4. **Experimental and Clinical Pharmacology of *Andrographis paniculata* and Its Major Bioactive Phytoconstituent Andrographolide**
5. ***Andrographis paniculata* in the Treatment of Upper Respira-**

tory Tract Infections: A Systematic Review of Safety and Efficacy

6. *Andrographis paniculata (Burm. f.) Wall. ex Nees: A Review of Ethnobotany, Phytochemistry, and Pharmacology*

19. Astragalus

1. Structural features and biological activities of the polysaccharides from Astragalus membranaceus.

2. Characterization of the Physiological Response following *In Vivo* Administration of *Astragalus membranaceus*

3. Modulatory Effects of *Astragalus* Polysaccharides on T-Cell Polarization in Mice with Polymicrobial Sepsis

4. Effect of Astragalus polysaccharides on expression of TNF-α, IL-1β and NFATc4 in a rat model of experimental colitis

5. *Astragalus* Oral Solution Ameliorates Allergic Asthma in Children by Regulating Relative Contents of CD4+CD25high-CD127low Treg Cells

20. Cat's Claw

1. Antiinflammatory actions of cat's claw: the role of NF−κB

2. Uncaria tomentosa aqueous-ethanol extract triggers an immunomodulation toward a Th2 cytokine profile.

3. Persistent response to pneumococcal vaccine in individuals supplemented with a novel water soluble extract of Uncaria tomentosa, C-Med-100.

21. Curcumin and Turmeric

1. Curcumin: A Review of Its' Effects on Human Health

2. Efficacy and safety of *Curcuma domestica* extracts compared with ibuprofen in patients with knee osteoarthritis: a multi-center study

3. Curcumin Suppresses the Alveolar Inflammation and Modulates the p53-Fibrinolytic System and Epithelial to Mesenchymal Transition During Lung Injury and Fibrosis In Vitro and In Vivo

4. Curcumin Suppression of Cytokine Release and Cytokine

Storm. A Potential Therapy for Patients with Ebola and Other Severe Viral Infections

5. Curcumin Suppression of Cytokine Release and Cytokine Storm. A Potential Therapy for Patients with Ebola and Other Severe Viral Infections

6. Curcumin: A Review of Its' Effects on Human Health

22. Echinacea

1. Echinacea-induced cytokine production by human macrophages.

2. Cytokine- and Interferon-Modulating Properties of *Echinacea* spp. Root Tinctures Stored at −20°C for 2 Years

3. Echinacea for upper respiratory infection

4. A proprietary extract from the echinacea plant (Echinacea purpurea) enhances systemic immune response during a common cold.

5. Echinacea root extracts for the prevention of upper respiratory tract infections: a double-blind, placebo-controlled randomized trial.

6. *Echinacea* and anti-inflammatory cytokine responses: Results of a gene and protein array analysis

7. Induction of multiple pro-inflammatory cytokines by respiratory viruses and reversal by standardized *Echinacea*, a potent antiviral herbal extract

8. *Echinacea*-Induced Macrophage Activation

23. Elderberry

1. The effect of Sambucol, a black elderberry-based, natural product, on the production of human cytokines: I. Inflammatory cytokines.

2. Black elderberry extract attenuates inflammation and metabolic dysfunction in diet-induced obese mice

3. The effect of herbal remedies on the production of human inflammatory and anti-inflammatory cytokines.

4. Cardiovascular Disease Risk Biomarkers and Liver and Kidney Function Are Not Altered in Postmenopausal Women after Ingesting an Elderberry Extract Rich in Anthocyanins for 12 Weeks

5. Elderberry and Elderflower Extracts, Phenolic Compounds, and Metabolites and Their Effect on Complement, RAW 264.7 Macrophages and Dendritic Cells

24. Eucalyptus

1. Effect of Eucalyptus Oil Inhalation on Pain and Inflammatory Responses after Total Knee Replacement: A Randomized Clinical Trial
2. Immune-Modifying and Antimicrobial Effects of Eucalyptus Oil and Simple Inhalation Devices

25. Garlic

1. Immunomodulation and Anti-Inflammatory Effects of Garlic Compounds
2. Immunomodulation and Anti-Inflammatory Effects of Garlic Compounds
3. Garlic Revisited: Therapeutic For The Major Diseases Of Our Times?
4. Allium sativum (garlic) suppresses leukocyte inflammatory cytokine production in vitro: Potential therapeutic use in the treatment of inflammatory bowel disease
5. The effect of garlic tablet on pro-inflammatory cytokines in postmenopausal osteoporotic women: a randomized controlled clinical trial
6. Evaluating the effect of garlic extract on serum inflammatory markers of peritoneal dialysis patients: a randomized double-blind clinical trial study
7. Garlic for the common cold
8. Supplementation with aged garlic extract improves both NK and $\gamma\delta$-T cell function and reduces the severity of cold and flu symptoms: a randomized, double-blind, placebo-controlled nutrition intervention.
9. WHO: Dengue and severe dengue
10. Garlic Organosulfur Compounds Reduce Inflammation and Oxidative Stress during Dengue Virus Infection
11. Low Allicin Release from Garlic Supplements: a Major Problem Due to the Sensitivities of Alliinase Activity

26. Ginger

1. The Amazing and Mighty Ginger
2. Anti-Oxidative and Anti-Inflammatory Effects of Ginger in Health and Physical Activity: Review of Current Evidence
3. Influence of dietary ginger (Zingiber officinales Rosc) on antioxidant defense system in rat: comparison with ascorbic acid.
4. Anti-Oxidative and Anti-Inflammatory Effects of Ginger in Health and Physical Activity: Review of Current Evidence
5. Fresh ginger (Zingiber officinale) has anti-viral activity against human respiratory syncytial virus in human respiratory tract cell lines.
6. Anti-Oxidative and Anti-Inflammatory Effects of Ginger in Health and Physical Activity: Review of Current Evidence
7. Anti-Inflammatory Effects of *Zingiber Officinale* in Type 2 Diabetic Patients
8. Effect of Ginger Supplementation on Proinflammatory Cytokines in Older Patients with Osteoarthritis: Outcomes of a Randomized Controlled Clinical Trial.
9. The effect of Zingiber officinale R. rhizomes (ginger) on plasma pro-inflammatory cytokine levels in well-trained male endurance runners.

27. Ginseng

1. Short-term oral administration of ginseng extract induces type-1 cytokine production
2. The Effect of Red Ginseng Extract on Inflammatory Cytokines after Chemotherapy in Children
3. The Yin and Yang actions of North American ginseng root in modulating the immune function of macrophages

28. Goldenseal and Berberine

1. Goldenseal and the common cold: The antibiotic myth

29. Green Tea—EGCG

1. Nutritional Modulation of Immune Function: Analysis of Evidence, Mechanisms, and Clinical Relevance
2. Nutritional Modulation of Immune Function: Analysis of Evidence, Mechanisms, and Clinical Relevance
3. **An Update on the Health Benefits of Green Tea**
4. **An Update on the Health Benefits of Green Tea**
5. **An Update on the Health Benefits of Green Tea**
6. EGCG In Green Tea Is Powerful Medicine Against Severe Sepsis, Lab Study Suggests
7. **A Major Ingredient of Green Tea Rescues Mice from Lethal Sepsis Partly by Inhibiting HMGB1**
8. **Green tea polyphenols change the profile of inflammatory cytokine release from lymphocytes of obese and lean rats and protect against oxidative damage.**
9. **Green tea with a high catechin content suppresses inflammatory cytokine expression in the galactosamine-injured rat liver.**
10. Effects of a 6-month green and black tea intervention on inflammatory cytokines: Role of gender and smoking

30. Licorice

1. **Licorice abuse: time to send a warning message**
2. Licorice
3. Is Licorice anti-viral?

31. Lomatium

1. Antiviral screening of British Columbian medicinal plants
2. Lomatium is not a broad spectrum "antiviral"

32. Milk Thistle

1. **Silymarin Inhibits In Vitro T-Cell Proliferation and Cytokine Production in Hepatitis C Virus Infection**
2. **Silibinin alleviates inflammation and induces apoptosis in**

human rheumatoid arthritis fibroblast-like synoviocytes and has a therapeutic effect on arthritis in rats

3. Immunostimulatory effect of Silybum Marianum (milk thistle) extract.
4. Immunosuppressive effect of silymarin on mitogen-activated protein kinase signalling pathway: the impact on T cell proliferation and cytokine production.
5. Silymarin Inhibits In Vitro T-Cell Proliferation and Cytokine Production in Hepatitis C Virus Infection
6. Silymarin improved diet-induced liver damage and insulin resistance by decreasing inflammation in mice
7. "Silymarin", a Promising Pharmacological Agent for Treatment of Diseases
8. Randomized controlled trial of silymarin treatment in patients with cirrhosis of the liver.
9. Effect of Silibinin on Humoral Immunology in Patients with Chronic Hepatitis C (This is a link to the google search that brought up this study. This study is the second hit. I'm including it because the actual link is a pdf download link and I have not been able to extract it from the google page.)

33. Olive Leaf

1. Oleuropein in Olive and its Pharmacological Effects
2. Impact of phenolic-rich olive leaf extract on blood pressure, plasma lipids and inflammatory markers: a randomised controlled trial
3. Human Intervention Study to Assess the Effects of Supplementation with Olive Leaf Extract on Peripheral Blood Mononuclear Cell Gene Expression
4. The effect of olive leaf extract in decreasing the expression of two pro-inflammatory cytokines in patients receiving chemotherapy for cancer. A randomized clinical trial.
5. The Effect of Olive Leaf Extract on Upper Respiratory Illness in High School Athletes: A Randomised Control Trial

34. Oregano

1. Effects of a combination of thyme and oregano essential oils on TNBS-induced colitis in mice.
2. Oregano Essential Oil Attenuates RAW264.7 Cells from Lipopolysaccharide-Induced Inflammatory Response through Regulating NADPH Oxidase Activation-Driven Oxidative Stress
3. Supercritical fluid extraction of oregano (*Origanum vulgare*) essentials oils: Anti-inflammatory properties based on cytokine response on THP-1 macrophages
4. Bactericidal Property of Oregano Oil Against Multidrug-Resistant Clinical Isolates
5. Antifungal activities of origanum oil against Candida albicans
6. Effects of Essential Oils and Monolaurin on *Staphylococcus aureus*: *In Vitro* and *In Vivo* Studies
7. Bactericidal Property of Oregano Oil Against Multidrug-Resistant Clinical Isolates

35. OSHA

1. http://www.jcimjournal.com/CN/abstract/abstract2136.shtml

36. Peppermint

1. In vitro antiviral, anti-inflammatory, and antioxidant activities of the ethanol extract of *Mentha piperita* L.

37. Red Clover

1. The effect of red clover isoflavones on menopausal symptoms, lipids and vaginal cytology in menopausal women: a randomized, double-blind, placebo-controlled study.
2. Intake of Novel Red Clover Supplementation for 12 Weeks Improves Bone Status in Healthy Menopausal Women
3. Effects of red clover on hot flash and circulating hormone concentrations in menopausal women: a systematic review and meta-analysis

4. Biochanin A inhibits lipopolysaccharide-induced inflammatory cytokines and mediators production in BV2 microglia.

38. St John's Wort

1. St. John's wort (Hypericum perforatum) counteracts cytokine-induced tryptophan catabolism in vitro.
2. Hyperforin, an anti-inflammatory constituent from St. John's wort, inhibits microsomal prostaglandin E2 synthase-1 and suppresses prostaglandin E2 formation *in vivo*
3. St. John's wort extract and hyperforin inhibit multiple phosphorylation steps of cytokine signaling and prevent inflammatory and apoptotic gene induction in pancreatic β cells
4. Hyperforin, an anti-inflammatory constituent from St. John's wort, inhibits microsomal prostaglandin E2 synthase-1 and suppresses prostaglandin E2 formation *in vivo*
5. St. John's Wort

CPSIA information can be obtained
at www.ICGtesting.com
Printed in the USA
FSHW011712120620

9 780984 190713